"How to create a moment in history. How to describe a journey from conception to birth with the moments of challenge, despair, humour and elation. Unique in this country.

Richard Smith likes an expedition, and this was truly an expedition. The book describes the dogged determination of this clinician surrounding himself with trusted experts, and that collective never giving up. It has been epic. The book is a fascinating read, carefully constructed, honest and open as I know my friend Richard to be.

As with natural conception, any complex and tortuous journey pales into insignificance with the inspirational end result."

Alan Farthing CVO, Consultant Gynaecologist,
Imperial College Healthcare NHS Trust and
King Edward VII Hospital London, UK

"The surgeons behind the UK's first womb transplant give unparalleled insight into the science, ethics, and teamwork that brought this important procedure to life. This book not only celebrates a remarkable medical achievement but also weaves a deeply human story of hope, resilience, and the power of collaboration."

Professor Nadey Hakim,
Imperial College London and
President-Elect, The Transplantation Society, UK

THE FIRST WOMB
TRANSPLANT IN THE UK

An Epic Journey to Motherhood

THE FIRST WOMB TRANSPLANT IN THE UK

An Epic Journey to Motherhood

J Richard Smith

Hammersmith and Queen Charlotte's and Chelsea Hospitals,
Imperial College Healthcare NHS Trust, UK

Isabel Quiroga-Giraldez

Churchill Hospital, Oxford University Hospitals NHS Foundation Trust, UK

Benjamin Jones

Lister Fertility Clinic, The Lister Hospital, UK

World Scientific

NEW JERSEY · LONDON · SINGAPORE · BEIJING · SHANGHAI · TAIPEI · CHENNAI

Published by

World Scientific Publishing Europe Ltd.

57 Shelton Street, Covent Garden, London WC2H 9HE

Head office: 5 Toh Tuck Link, Singapore 596224

USA office: 27 Warren Street, Suite 401-402, Hackensack, NJ 07601

Library of Congress Control Number: 2025008594

British Library Cataloguing-in-Publication Data
A catalogue record for this book is available from the British Library.

A percentage of royalties will be donated to Womb Transplant UK, charity number 1138559.

THE FIRST WOMB TRANSPLANT IN THE UK
An Epic Journey to Motherhood

ISBN 978-1-80061-770-4 (hardcover)
ISBN 978-1-80061-776-6 (paperback)
ISBN 978-1-80061-771-1 (ebook for institutions)
ISBN 978-1-80061-772-8 (ebook for individuals)

For any available supplementary material, please visit
https://www.worldscientific.com/worldscibooks/10.1142/Q0522#t=suppl

Desk Editors: Aanand Jayaraman/Rosie Williamson

Typeset by Stallion Press
Email: enquiries@stallionpress.com

Success is not final, failure is not fatal: it is the courage to continue that counts.

WS Churchill

Dedication

J Richard Smith: To the first wonderful family to emerge from Womb Transplant UK: Grace, Angus and baby Amy Isabel, and to those who will hopefully follow them. Thank you for your patience, bravery and resilience, and for trusting us through many trials and tribulations. Also I dedicate this book to my dearest friend Isabel for her belief in the project and her consummate surgical and oratorical ability; to Ben, my brother in arms, for his powers of advocacy and tenacity; to Srdjan, who provided a bedrock; to Sal and Ari, for their perseverance and dedication to the cause; to Bryony, Charlie, Clare and Paul, who so skilfully managed Grace's pregnancy and delivery; and to the whole extended team for their huge effort over many years to allow this project to come to fruition.

Finally, I dedicate this book to my family: to my children, Cameron, Victoria, Madeleine and Lara, and to my mother Diana and sister Alison, who have provided the foundations to allow me to thrive and hold on.

Isabel Quiroga-Giraldez: To baby Amy Isabel and her parents, Grace and Angus; I am deeply honoured and touched that my name became hers. To Andrea, with my deepest gratitude for all the hours of effort to propel this project over the line. To Clare, who is the rock of the project, caring for our patients and linking us all. To Venkatesha and Ann, for providing the much-needed support during this arduous surgery, and to my Oxford friends and colleagues for all of their wise counsel, assistance and unbelievable effort.

At the London end of this project, to my dear friend, surgical partner, co-lecturer and collaborator Richard, who has held us all together as we have become one joint uterine transplant team across two cities: not always an easy process, but a great strength. To Bryony, who invited me to be at the delivery — I was thrilled to be present at such a special moment. To Neil Huband, who has given me so much valued advice with respect to the media, without which we might have been engulfed.

Finally, I dedicate this book, with my greatest thanks, to my parents, my sister, nephew, niece, and extended family for their lifelong support and love, and to my wonderful son Jaime, for all his love and caring.

This project has been a stressful but wonderful journey to offer hope to many women who previously had none, and I am so glad to have been part of it.

Benjamin Jones: To Grace, your trust, courage, and belief in our team made this possible and has now paved the way for countless others. Your strength in facing the unknown and refusal to give up have forever changed the possibilities of medicine and motherhood. Your legacy will now inspire many generations to come. To Angus, you have always stood as a pillar of strength throughout. Your steadfast support and patience have always brought balance and composure to the most difficult of situations! To Amy, the sister whose love knew no bounds! Your generosity and kindness truly encompass the real meaning of family.

To Richard, working with you has been an honour and a privilege. Your leadership and dedication continue to inspire! To my incredible colleagues at the Lister Fertility Clinic, you played a vital role in this groundbreaking journey, bringing hope and new beginnings to those who dare to dream. Thank you for making miracles happen every day!

Finally, to my beloved Claire, and children Scarlett and Lucius. You are my greatest inspiration and the driving force behind everything I do. Your love, laughter, and unwavering support give my life purpose and joy. Every day, you remind me of what truly matters, and for that, I am endlessly grateful.

Foreword by the Baroness Cox

It gives me great pleasure to write a Foreword for this book, which tells the 25-year story of the effort in the UK to give comfort to women suffering from infertility — having been born without a womb, having lost their womb due to hysterectomy, or having a non-functioning womb.

This book takes the reader through this story with its up and downs, successes and failures. It follows the invention of procedures that have allowed fertility to be preserved whilst treating cancer and other conditions that used to invariably result in hysterectomy. A number of world-firsts in the fields of infertility and gynaecological cancer management are described here.

The team have shared their commitments, through many challenges, to deliver a uterine transplant programme for the women of the UK, which will bring hope to many for whom there previously was no effective solution.

A percentage of royalties from this book go to the charity Womb Transplant UK, of which I am a Patron; the charity currently has funds for two more procedures, and I would urge you to go to their website (https://wombtransplantuk.org/) if you wish to donate to enable the practice of more of these life-changing procedures.

Table of Contents

Part I: Transplant History

Part II: Early Days of Fertility Preservation and Restoration

Part III: Progress and Surgery

Part IV: Future Research and Considerations

Acknowledgements

Surgeons and gynaecologists supporting the early work: Mr David Corless, Dr Giuseppe Del Priore, Mr Faris Zakaria, Miss Deborah Boyle, Mr Krishen Sieunarine, and Mr Paul Moxey

Academic surgical supporters: Professors Sadaf Ghaem-Maghami, Peter Friend, Stephen Kennedy, Rutger Ploeg, Jane Blazeby, and Mr Sanjay Sinha

Tissue engineering: Professor Dame Molly Stevens DBE FRS

Royal Veterinary College: Professor David Noakes and Dr Michael Boyd

Law and ethics: Professors Stephen Wilkinson (Lancaster University) and Amel Alghrani (University of Liverpool) and Dr Natasha Hammond-Browning (Cardiff University)

Public relations and publishing, Womb Transplant UK: Mr Neil Huband and Mr John Harrison

Public relations, Imperial College London: Piers Wright

Public relations, Oxford University Hospitals (OUH): Roy Probert

Tour managers: Ed Smith and Hamish Pirie

Publisher: Laurent Chaminade

Advanced haemostasis practitioner: Antonio Barbosa

Porters: Nigel Spencer, Fiaz Saddiq, and Zia Murtaza

Senior OUH managers: Professor Chris Cunningham and Mr Rainer Buhler

Transplant colleagues: Professors Peter Friend, Rutger Ploeg, Messrs Sanjay Sinha, and Srikanth Reddy

Virology: Professor Katie Jeffery

Transplant Immunology Laboratory: Drs Martin Barnardo, Jeanette Ayers, and Mian Chen

Current PhD Fellows: Dr Saaliha Vali and Dr Ariadne L'Heveder

Radiology, psychology and histopathology: Dr Victoria Stewart, Dr Nishat Bharwani, Professor Anna David, Dr Maria Jalmbrant, Dr Alex Clarke, Dr Ian Lindsay, Dr Baljeet Kaur, Dr Candice Roufosse, and Dr Louise Hankinson

Early Pregnancy and MRKH Unit at Queen Charlotte's and Chelsea Hospital: Miss Maya Al-Memar and Sr Margaret Campbell

Obstetrics: Miss Bryony Jones and Dr Charlotte Frise

Uterine transplant team: Professor J Richard Smith, Miss Isabel Quiroga-Giraldez, Mr Ben Jones, Dr Saaliha Vali, Mr Venkatesha Udupa, Mr Srdjan Saso, Miss Ann Ogbemudia, Miss Sushma Shankar, Mr Keno Mentor, Miss Irene Mosca, Professor Sadaf Ghaem-Maghami, Dr Cesar Diaz-Garcia, Mr Ahmad Sayasneh, and Professor Jay Chatterjee

Our collaborators at Baylor University Medical Center, Dallas, USA: Drs Liza Johannesson and Giuliano Testa

JR Smith would also like to thank Petroula and Kostos Stergiou for their wonderful hospitality at the Petra Hotel, Grikos, on the Isle of Patmos. Much of this book was written in that wonderfully inspiring place. Also, many thanks to Yiorgos, Gerty and Christina Moraiti, and to Christina's husband Tassos Koutsevelis and their son Vasilios in Kioni, Ithaki, for their support and help in printing earlier drafts; the studio, print facilities and friendship there were vital to the process. He would also like to thank Catrina Donegan, his sister Alison and his now-grown-up children for 'minding the fort' whilst he has been away on these trips.

In addition, we would all like to thank the Cotswold Lodge Hotel in Oxford for the warm welcome and comfortable surroundings, with some of the final editing of this book taking place in their drawing room.

The Authors

J Richard Smith, MB ChB, MD, DSc, FRCOG

Consultant Gynaecological Surgeon, Hammersmith and Queen Charlotte's and Chelsea Hospitals, Imperial College Healthcare NHS Trust, London, UK

Professor of Practice, Imperial College London, UK

Adjunct Associate Professor of Gynecology (1995–2020), New York University Medical Center, New York, USA

Honorary Consultant in Transplantation Surgery, Churchill Hospital, Oxford University Hospitals NHS Foundation Trust, Oxford, UK

Professor J Richard Smith trained as a doctor in Glasgow (1977–1982) and in London, obtaining his MRCOG in 1988 and graduating with an MD from the University of Glasgow on cervical cancer, immunity and infection in 1992. In 2023, he was awarded a DSc by the University of Glasgow for his submitted thesis by publication entitled 'Fertility Preservation and Restoration.' In the 1990s, he worked as a lecturer and senior lecturer at Charing Cross and Westminster Medical School. He then became Director of Gynaecology at Chelsea and Westminster Hospital and a visiting associate professor at NYU Medical Center in New York. Since 2005, he has been based at the West London Gynaecological Cancer Centre, Hammersmith and Queen Charlotte's and Chelsea Hospitals, Imperial College Healthcare NHS Trust. He was an adjunct associate professor at NYU Medical Center from 1995 to 2020. He is a Professor of Practice at Imperial College London and an Honorary Consultant in Transplantation Surgery at Oxford University Hospitals. He is the founder and chair of the charity Womb Transplant UK and leader of the research team – a project he has been involved with for the past 25 years.

Miss Isabel Quiroga-Giraldez, LMS, MSc, DPhil, FRCS

Consultant in Transplantation and Endocrine Surgery, Churchill Hospital, Oxford University Hospitals NHS Foundation Trust, Oxford, UK

Honorary Consultant Gynaecological Surgeon, Hammersmith and Queen Charlotte's and Chelsea Hospitals, Imperial College Healthcare NHS Trust, London, UK

Miss Isabel Quiroga-Giraldez graduated from the Universidad Complutense de Madrid, Spain, in 1993 with an MSc in Humanitarian Medicine. She moved to Oxford in 1999, graduating with a DPhil (Oxon) in 2004. She has been a key member of the Womb Transplant UK team since 2014, involved with all aspects of both uterine and endometrial transplantation work. Her principal work is in the field of renal and pancreatic transplant surgery, of which she is the clinical lead for organ retrieval. She is also co-leader of the uterine transplant, leading the implantation procedures. She has brought to the team her impressive transplant skills in the field of microsurgery and her knowledge of managing immunosuppressed transplant patients.

Mr Benjamin Jones, MBChB, BSc (Hons), PhD, MRCOG

Consultant Gynaecologist and Fertility Specialist, Lister Fertility Clinic, the Lister Hospital, London, UK

Honorary Consultant Gynaecologist, Imperial College Healthcare NHS Trust, London, UK

Honorary Consultant in Transplantation Surgery, Oxford Transplant Centre, Oxford University Hospitals NHS Foundation Trust, Oxford, UK

Honorary Clinical Lecturer, Faculty of Medicine, Department of Metabolism, Digestion and Reproduction, Institute of Reproductive & Developmental Biology, Hammersmith Hospital Campus, Imperial College London, London, UK

Mr Benjamin Jones graduated from the University of Leeds in 2009. His BSc (Hons) was in sports science in relation to medicine. He obtained his MRCOG in 2015 and graduated with a PhD from Imperial College in 2021. His PhD was on fertility preservation and restoration, including uterine transplantation, endometrial transplantation and elective oocyte cryopreservation. He is the coordinator and co-leader of both programmes and is trained in gynaecological surgery and infertility. He is a consultant gynaecologist and fertility specialist at the Lister Hospital, London.

The Team

Throughout the book, the team members will be referred to by their first names. The following includes a short CV for each of them. All members of the team have given freely of their time and effort over many years.

One of the amazing things about the team is their confluence of surgical skills; gynaecological cancer surgery and transplant surgery are like a Venn diagram, with much overlap but also quite different mixes of skills. The cancer surgeon aims to remove a diseased organ to send it in for analysis. This involves sealing and occluding its blood supply with a margin of normal tissue around the tumour. The transplant surgeon removes a healthy organ with no margin of normal tissue to put into another patient. This requires vessels to be intact and suitable to suture into the recipient. This juxtaposition of skills is essential in uterine transplantation, and thus, the team members as constituted are dependent on one another for a successful outcome.

Professor J Richard Smith is a Consultant Gynaecological Surgeon at Hammersmith and Queen Charlotte's and Chelsea Hospitals, Imperial College Healthcare NHS Trust. He is the Chief Investigator of the deceased donor programme and co-lead surgeon for the living donor programme, focusing on uterus retrieval.

Miss Isabel Quiroga-Giraldez is a Consultant in Transplantation and Endocrine Surgery at the Oxford Transplant Centre. She is the co-lead surgeon for the living donor programme, focussing on uterine implantation, and the Principal Investigator at Oxford University Hospitals NHS Foundation Trust for the deceased donor programme.

Mr Benjamin Jones is a Consultant Gynaecologist and Fertility Specialist at Lister Fertility Clinic. He orchestrated the transition from research concept in animal models to surgical procedure in women in the UK. He coordinates the living and deceased donor programmes and is the Principal Investigator for the deceased donor programme at Imperial College Healthcare NHS Trust.

Mr Venkatesha Udupa is a Consultant in Transplantation and Hepatobiliary Surgery at Oxford University Hospitals, specialising in renal, pancreatic and gastrointestinal transplant surgery. He is involved in the surgery and ongoing management of all the patients.

Mr Srdjan Saso is a Consultant Gynaecological Oncologist at Hammersmith and Queen Charlotte's and Chelsea Hospitals, Imperial College Healthcare NHS Trust. He completed a PhD at Imperial College London focused on the general surgical aspects of fertility preservation and the anatomical, immunological and psychological issues related to uterine transplantation.

Dr Saaliha (Sal) Vali is a PhD student at Imperial College London who has been assiduous and vital in bringing the programme to its conclusion.

Dr Ariadne (Ari) L'Heveder is an Honorary Research Fellow at Imperial College London. An obstetrician at heart, she has joined the programme at just the point where those skills will be needed.

Dr Andrea Devaney is the Lead Pharmacist in Transplantation and Renal Services at the Oxford Transplant Centre. She has been a tower of support to the uterine transplant programme, writing protocols, attending committees and imparting much clinical advice.

Miss Ann Ogbemudia is a Specialist Registrar in General Surgery and Transplantation at the Oxford Deanery. She partakes in all the surgeries and ongoing care of the patients.

Professor Yau Thum is a Fertility Specialist at the Lister Fertility Clinic, London. As our infertility lead, Yau has brought an encyclopaedic knowledge of infertility and IVF to the team.

Dr Timothy Bracewell-Milnes is a Consultant Gynaecologist and Subspecialist in Reproductive Medicine and Surgery at the Lister Fertility Clinic. He has also contributed much over many years.

Dr Maria Jalmbrant (Sloane Court Clinic, London), **Dr Alex Clarke** (Royal Free Hospital, London) and **Dr Louise Hankinson** (Churchill Hospital, Oxford) are our psychological advisors.

Dr Neil Clancy is a Junior Research Fellow in the Department of Surgery and Cancer and the Hamlyn Centre for Medical Robotics at Imperial College London.

Dr Maxine Chan is an Obstetrician and Gynecologist. She obtained her PhD in Tissue Engineering in the laboratories of Professor Dame Molly Stevens at Imperial College London.

Professor Sadaf Ghaem-Maghami (Imperial College London), **Mr Ahmad Sayasneh** (St Thomas' Hospital, London) and **Professor Jay Chatterjee** (Royal Surrey Hospital NHS Foundation Trust, Guildford) are Gynaecological Oncologic Surgeons who are 'ticketed' as organ retrievers with NHS Blood and Transplant for deceased organ donation. The same applies to **Dr Cesar Diaz-Garcia** (Glasgow Clinical Research Facility), an Oncological Surgeon, infertility specialist and an original member of the Swedish Uterine Transplant programme.

Dr Paul Harding is a Consultant Nephrologist at Oxford University Hospitals. He advises this group with respect to kidney function in prospective patients and supporting the transplanted patients.

Professor Katie Jeffery is a Consultant Virologist at Oxford University Hospitals. She advises this group with respect to viruses such as cytomegalovirus (CMV), Epstein-Barr virus (EBV), and the like.

Drs Martin Barnardo, Jeanette Ayers, and **Mian Chen** look after transplant immunology at Oxford University Hospitals.

Drs Peter Dimitrov, Andris Klucniks, Richard Katz, and **Lee Yee Tee** are Consultant Anaesthetists at Oxford University Hospitals. They work with us for all the uterine transplants at Oxford University Hospitals.

Miss Bryony Jones is a Consultant at Queen Charlotte's and Chelsea Hospital, London. She specialises in high-risk obstetrics and is caring for the patients during pregnancy.

Miss Maya Al-Memar is a Consultant at Queen Charlotte's and Chelsea Hospital, London. She specialises in early pregnancy and leads the Mayer-Rokitansky-Küster-Hauser syndrome (MRKH) Unit.

Sr Margaret Campbell is a Senior Specialist Nurse at the Mayer-Rokitansky-Küster-Hauser syndrome (MRKH) Unit, Queen Charlotte's and Chelsea Hospital, London.

Drs Baljeet Kaur, Candice Roufosse and **Ian Lindsay** (Imperial College London) have performed all the histopathology over many years.

Mr Neil Huband (Priority Council) has provided public relations and media support to Womb Transplant UK over the course of two decades, gratis.

Professor David Noakes and **Dr Michael Boyd** at the Royal Veterinary College were the key veterinarian professionals in the original porcine, rabbit and sheep projects.

Professor Francis Jimenez is a Professor of Veterinarian Medicine at Universitat Politècnica de València, Spain, who brought the original rabbit embryos to London and more recently has held the Project License for the endometrial transplant research.

Dr Giuseppe Del Priore is a Professor of Gynaecologic Oncology at Grady Memorial Hospital, Atlanta, USA, and our long-term US friend and collaborator.

Mr David Corless is a Consultant in General Surgery at Mid Cheshire Hospitals NHS Foundation Trust and supported this project from its inception.

Notes on the Text

Confidentiality

Patient confidentiality is a time-honoured principle of medical ethics. The patients referred to in this book have given permission for their medical histories to be published. Only names and other identifying details have been altered in order to protect their privacy. Their stories are true and inspiring.

The Derivation of Gynaecological Words

Gynaecology is unusual amongst the medical specialities in that most organs have two names – one Greek derived, the other Latin. *Hysteros*, Greek for womb, is *uterus* in Latin; *colpos*, Greek for 'blind-ending sac,' is *vagina* in Latin. Following the same pattern is *oophoros* from Greek, meaning 'egg-bearing,' and *ovarium* (plural *ovaria*), or ovary, from the Latin; *trachelos*, the Greek for 'neck,' is the equivalent of *cervix*, or the 'neck' of the womb. Finally, to break all the rules, there is the Fallopian tube, named after an Italian anatomist, Gabriello Fallopio. Removal of the Fallopian tube is called salpingectomy, again derived from the Greek word for the Fallopian tube, *salpinx* (derived from a trumpet-like instrument of the Ancient Greeks). As you may have noticed, if we refer to the organ itself, it is in its Latin form, but for procedures to be performed, we use the Greek name of the organ – e.g., to remove the uterus is a hysterectomy.

List of Acronyms

APSN   atypical placental site nodules (form of GTD)

ART   abdominal radical trachelectomy

AUFI   absolute uterine factor infertility

BMI   body mass index

CIN   cervical intraepithelial neoplasia

CMV   cytomegalovirus

DBD   donation after brainstem death

ECM   extra cellular matrix

ETT   embryonic trophoblastic tumour (form of GTD)

FS   frozen section

GTD   gestational trophoblastic disease

HCA   healthcare assistant

HPV   human papillomavirus

HTA   Human Tissue Authority

ITU   intensive care unit

IVF   *in vitro* fertilisation

LD   living donors

MDT   multidisciplinary team

MFAT	microfragmented adipose fat
MRKH	Mayer-Rokitansky-Küster-Hauser syndrome
NHSBT	NHS Blood and Transplantation
NODC	National Organ Donation Committee
NRG	National Retrieval Group
PRP	protein rich plasma
PSTT	placental site trophoblastic tumour (form of GTD)
RCOG	Royal College of Obstetricians and Gynaecologists
RI	Royal Institution
SIL	squamous intraepithelial lesion (American equivalent word for CIN)
SNOD	specialist nurses in organ donation
UTx	uterine transplant
VAPs	vasoactive peptides
VIN	vulval intraepithelial neoplasia

Introduction

We had obtained ethics approval and appeared to be on the brink of performing uterine transplants in the UK in 2015, when we were first approached by Imperial College Press (now World Scientific Publishing Europe) to put this book together. Little did we realise the tortuous path of regulatory processes we still had to follow. And then January 2020 arrived. We had all the necessary permissions in place, and our on-call rota for deceased donors went live. The team were called six times in January and February of 2020, but on three occasions the donors were unsuitable, and on the other three the families did not wish any organs to be donated, meaning that we were stood down.

Our living donor programme was just at the point of 'lift-off' when COVID-19 arrived on the scene. Literally, the first UK live donor transplant was booked for 22nd March 2020, the day before lockdown was formally announced in the UK. We had no option but to cancel the procedure. COVID-19 had also impacted our practice runs: one scheduled for 12th March couldn't happen because Isabel was sick, and it turned out, by the 13th, that the patient had contracted COVID-19. Richard and most of his surgical team were down with COVID-19 themselves, courtesy of the practise run itself. By 22nd March, Richard was in hospital on oxygen going downhill fast; wills were being signed! It's fair to say that the planets were not aligned.

Happily, everyone recovered, and Richard and team were alive and kicking, with the transplant programmes, both living and deceased, now underway. After the worst of the pandemic, it then took two years of meetings, much cajoling, and many joint efforts to get both programmes to the point of restart. It is easy to forget that amid all of these frustrations, our patients and their partners had been put through hell, we are very sorry to say. But meeting these couples proved to be our driver to never give up.

This book is a genuine tale of scientific and surgical exploration, recounting the stories of the many participants who have brought this project to fruition with a dual programme of living donors (LD) and donation after brainstem death (DBD). A huge number of people have contributed to this project over the years, as can be seen in the acknowledgements and the team members; this has genuinely been a decades-long team effort. The patients have been unbelievably patient with us and the myriad of delays that have dogged this project.

Anyway, here it is: our story, warts and all — a long-term surgical and scientific research programme that has had many successes and not a few failures. We have deliberately written in a chatty style, and the narrative is largely recounted from Richard's point of view for simplicity and continuity. However, as with the transplant itself, the writing of this book has been a team effort, with invaluable input from Isabel and Ben. Moreover, some sections focus on topics that different uterine transplant team members have written on and published in academic scientific journals. For those who are interested, our group has amassed approximately 120 peer-reviewed publications on these topics, and these are referenced on pages 175 to 189, with the papers themselves available on PubMed.

Who Wants a Uterine Transplant?

The simple answer is 'women with absolute uterine factor infertility who wish to have a baby.' However, as you might imagine, it's not quite so simple as that. Absolute uterine factor infertility is, by defini-tion, where a woman has no uterus, or has a uterus incapable of repro-duction. Other options exist for treatment by way of adoption and surrogacy. Adoption is well established but bureaucratically difficult. It is, however, safe for mother and child and, socially, it has the advantage of allowing children with no parental support a family to be brought up in. Of course, its downside is lack of genetic transference and the difficulties that may arise from this for both the parents and the children.

Surrogacy is performed in the UK 400–500 times per year. In surrogacy, eggs are taken from the putative mother mixed with her partner's sperm, and an embryo is created by IVF. The embryo is then implanted into the surrogate. In the UK, this would be an altruistic volunteer woman, who is unpaid excepting her expenses. The surrogate mother delivers the baby, and the baby is legally adopted by the genetic parents. This is an arrangement that works well in that it allows women with no womb to have a child that is genetically their own.

The disadvantages are that there are several concerns for the genetic parents until the process is complete. Legally, the surrogate mother could refuse to allow the baby to be adopted; this very rarely happens, but it is a cause of anxiety until the paperwork is formally signed. In addition, there are issues for many genetic mothers relating to their desire to carry a pregnancy and give birth.

Furthermore, in our experience, genetic mothers worry much about what the surrogate is eating and drinking during the pregnancy, which is entirely out of the genetic mother's control. These factors are further compounded by social differences between the genetic and surrogate mothers. In countries where the surrogate mothers are paid, these issues can multiply. A colleague of ours in America related the story of a surrogate mother in the Midwest who went into premature labour with premature rupture of the membranes containing amniotic fluid. This puts both the mother and baby at risk of infection, but of course, delivery also means the baby will be premature. Meanwhile, the genetic mother, based in New York, harangued the obstetrician to not deliver the baby prematurely and threatened not to follow through with the process of paying the surrogate or accepting the baby if not in good condition – a complex situation, we are sure you will agree.

This is where uterine transplantation, for all its difficulties, does solve many problems. In uterine transplantation, a woman is able to carry her own genetically related baby and deliver it, albeit by Caesarean section.

The Causes of Absolute Uterine Factor Infertility

It is estimated that there are 50,000 women in the UK with absolute uterine factor infertility. The principal group are women who have been born without, or with only a vestige, of a uterus. The women will have ovaries, but while some have a normal-length vagina, others have one that is shorter in length. This condition is called Mayer-Rokitansky-Küster-Hauser Syndrome, and it affects every 1 in 4,000 to 5,000 women, meaning that it will affect around 5,000 women in the UK of reproductive age at any given time. The majority of women who have approached us regarding a uterine transplant have this condition.

Other reasons for absolute uterine factor infertility include women who have had hysterectomies (otherwise known as the removal of the uterus) for haemorrhage and cancer. Modern advances in treatment mean that it is less common for cervical cancer to require hysterectomy. However, gestational trophoblastic disease (GTD), cancer of the placenta (afterbirth), sarcomatous tumours of the uterus, and cancer of the endometrium are all treated using this procedure. The last of these cancers is becoming increasingly common in young women due to of increasing rates of obesity, and unless found at an early stage, it requires treatment by hysterectomy. Cervical cancer now less commonly requires hysterectomy, and this will be discussed in greater detail later in this book. Of all the women who have approached us, only a few have had cancer whereby they lost their uterus.

The final group are those women who have a uterus, but one that is non-functioning. Reasons for this might include lacking a suitable lining to the uterus or the endometrium; Asherman's syndrome (also to be discussed later); massive fibroids (benign growths in the uterus); adenomyosis (where the endometrium has implanted in the muscle of the uterus); and severe endometriosis that makes the uterus incapable of reproduction.

Ethics

This book describes many research projects, including human- and animal-based projects, all of which have had appropriate Ethics Committee approvals prior to being undertaken. All human projects went through independent Ethics Committees at the appropriate Institutions at the time. Animal-based works were performed at the Royal Veterinary College, London (RVC) and were all approved by the RVC Ethics Committee and were Home Office licensed. All those who took part held the correct Personal Licenses and had passed the appropriate examinations. Projects performed at the Universitat Politècnica de València were all Ethics-approved at that institution.

A conference for researchers on this subject was held in Indianapolis in December 2011 which was attended by Richard and Srdjan. It produced a consensus document laying out ethical guidelines for uterine transplant eligibility at that time. This created a set of criteria related to the evolving research.

Clearly, since then, much has moved on. In 2016, Richard and Ben attended a two-day conference on the ethics of uterine transplantation. It was here where we learned about the 2010 Gender Equality Act, which mandates equal care, if technically feasible, for transgender and women assigned male at birth. This will be discussed in greater detail in Chapter 12.

Animal-based research is contentious. However, the nature of our research meant that this sort of research was essential, and the small number of animals involved have greatly contributed to the advance of gynaecological surgery. All of the animals used in this research were cared for very well, with temperature, lighting and noise levels optimally controlled to keep the animals comfortable. They had access to ample food and water and were appropriately housed, without overcrowding and with adequate bedding. A much wider discussion on the ethics of uterine transplantation can be found in Chapter 11.

The Charity

The Womb Transplant UK charity (No. 1138559) was set up in 2010 to do what it says on the tin: to fund research into womb transplantation, and to allow the first ten deceased donor transplant and first five living donor transplants to be performed cost-neutral to the NHS. Richard is the chairman of the charity, and a portion of royalties from this book will be donated to Womb Transplant UK.

The charity was born out of a conversation with a patient who happened to be a chief fundraiser for a major institution. Having sorted her medical issues, I asked her advice on how to obtain funding for my research into womb transplantation, somewhere in the region of £250,000–500,000. I was really struggling to obtain any funding! To this, she said, 'That's nothing; there are plenty of people who will sit in this seat [the one she was sitting on] to whom that is like flicking a coin in a fountain; the trouble is you can't ask them!' I agreed wholeheartedly. She instead recommended establishing a charity, commenting that 'You will probably find that one individual decides to donate the lot.' Sadly, this has never happened, although we have seen some enormously generous donations, particularly from our new patrons Nick Maughan CBE and Nadine Kaneva, for whom we are all incredibly grateful.

I set up the charity through our family solicitor, Alan Levinson, with Mike Stafford and Tom Lewis (sadly now deceased) as trustees. This process was slow, primarily because George Osborne, Chancellor of the Exchequer at that time, was pretty resistant to new charities, but with Alan's drive, eventually Womb Transplant UK came into being. This was all new to me, but what we now required was a patron or two or three.

I first reached out to the remarkable Baroness Masham of Ilton (sadly deceased 2023), whom I had known for many years, and she graciously accepted. Sue was originally in the House of Lords as

Countess of Swinton and became a Baroness in her own right for all that she had achieved for the disabled community; she was a Paralympic medallist herself. The second Patron was Miss Kate Fitzsimmons (sadly deceased 2024), a retired Matron of St Mary's Hospital from back in the 1980s. She was another remarkable woman who knew how to 'control' Senior Consultants – a very particular skill. Kate also suggested that the Baroness Cox would make an excellent third Patron. Baroness Caroline Cox is a very special woman of enormous integrity and personal bravery. She goes to all those places the Foreign Office say to avoid – for example, North Korea and Northeast Africa – in pursuit of humanitarian aid. Like Sue, Caroline has done much to champion disability and was herself originally a nurse. She also hails from surgical royalty; she always tells doctors that her father was Robert J McNeill Love, of the very famous surgical textbook by Bailey and Love, a book that most of us have on our shelves. Kate and I duly wrote to Baroness Cox, but we didn't really get anywhere at the time; I had little idea just how busy she was. When, a few months later, Sue (Baroness Masham) discovered our lack of progress, she hosted an afternoon tea at the House of Lords so that we might meet Caroline, Baroness Cox.

A few weeks later, Tom Lewis and I duly ventured to the Palace of Westminster. When you arrive there, you know undoubtedly that you are at the centre of the 'hive.' John Prescott was exiting the foyer as we arrived. He was shorter than I had expected; I think that the episode where he punched the journalist (the one that raised his popularity) had led me to imagine a much larger guy. Once Tom and I were settled for afternoon tea, we were kindly offered biscuits or cake: I went for the biscuit. As it arrived, Sue lent forward and said, 'I think you should get on and eat that biscuit before Caroline arrives… when she gets here there won't be much time for biscuit-eating!'

Sure enough, once Baroness Cox had finished addressing the House, she approached to ask about our story: I accordingly gave her the ten-minute version of the womb transplant story. Caroline proceeded to ask very pertinent and penetrating questions for the next 40 minutes, and graciously agreed to become a Patron of the charity. Wow, what an afternoon! I will confess that Tom and I did a high-five once we had made our goodbyes and were safely around the corner. I had worn my best three-piece suit to tea; in fact, Tom had commented earlier that he hadn't seen it before, despite the fact that we had worked together for 10 years at that point and had been friends for 20. I opened up my jacket to show Tom that my shirt below the armpits was saturated in sweat. I had, however, passed this serious *viva voce*.

The charity now had three very special patrons, which has allowed us to host charity dinners at the House of Lords, sponsored by Caroline, and to raise the funds that have allowed us to continue. Our Patrons have been a genuine tower of support and encouragement through the years. We have also had some entertaining meetings in pursuit of funding: one included vying for the opportunity to give a lecture at C. Hoare and Co.'s bank philanthropy meetings. Another philanthropist at the table suggested that one of 'his scientists' — a Nobel laureate — could give a talk. I knew, at that point, that I was out of my depth! Sadly, I never did deliver that talk. However, courtesy of our patrons we have continued to slowly raise funds. The Kirby Laing Foundation and The Abdalla Foundation, and more recently our newest patrons Mr Nick Maughan CBE and Ms Nadine Kaneva, have been very generous to us. Many others have contributed both their time and their effort over the years running charitable events to support us.

I have also published three non-medical books, *The Journey: Spirituality, Pilgrimage, Chant* (Darton, Longman and Todd, 2016); *A Very Byzantine Journey* (Sacristy Press, 2022); and *The Monymusk Reliquary: The Brecbennach of St Columba* (JR Smith Healthcare, 2024). All royalties from these books, along with a percentage of this one and my other medical book *Women's Cancers: Pathways to Living* (Imperial College Press, 2015) go to the charity, so please do purchase for a good cause if you are interested.

• Part I •
Transplant History

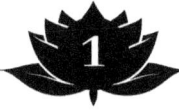

Transplants: A History

A General History of Transplants

Let's start by going back in time into the history of transplant surgery. Transplantation has been a dream of medical science for centuries. However, it was only in 1954 that the first successful kidney transplant took place; it was between identical twins, so no immunosuppressive therapy was required. Much later, with the advent of effective immuno-suppression, renal transplantation took off, which will be touched on in more detail later. In 1966, the first successful simultaneous kidney and pancreas transplant took place. This was followed in 1967, when Starzl performed the first liver transplant. 1968 saw the first life-saving transplant of the heart. Later, lung transplants followed.

These transplants were all life-saving. What follows is life-enhancing. The first hand transplant occurred in 1998. Face transplant followed in 2011. In 2000, the first unsuccessful uterine transplant took place. A further 14 years followed before a successful procedure was completed in Sweden. More recently, in 2023, an eye was transplanted.

It is the case in most transplants that there are about 10–15 years between first procedure to reasonable wider adoption. As with any new procedure, the development of the technical aspects and fine-tuning of the management take time. Vital in the arena of trans-plantation has been the concurrent development of new and more effective immunosuppressive treatments to prevent graft rejection. In addition, there is a requirement to bring colleagues — both medical and nursing — and the wider public on board with these developments which many regard initially as too risky or too expensive.

Taking pancreatic transplantation as an example, Figure 1.1 the following graph shows the very slow rise in pancreatic transplant numbers from the start in the 1970s, to real take-off by the mid to late 80s. Annual numbers then exponentially increased through the 90s to present-day levels.

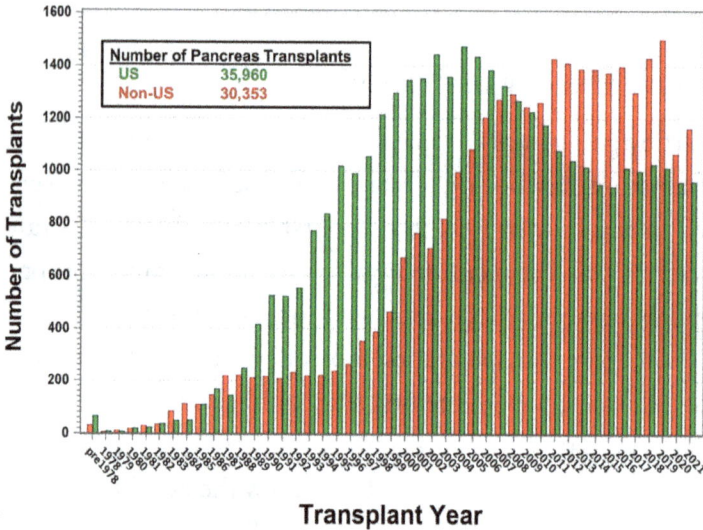

Figure 1.1. Number of pancreas transplants reported to the International Pancreas Transplant Registry (IPTR) between 17 December 1966 and 31 December 2021.

Source: Angelika C. Gruessner, "A Decade of Pancreas Transplantation — A Registry Report," Uro 3(2), 132–150, 2023. CC BY 4.0 (https://creativecommons.org/licenses/by/4.0/)

As the map in Figure 1.2 so aptly demonstrates, transplantation rates vary greatly, with geographical location with the United States and Spain leading the world in terms of transplant numbers. The total number of transplants worldwide in 2021 was 144,302, an 11.3% increase over 2020. There were 38,156 deceased donors donating various combinations of heart, lungs, kidneys, livers, pancreata, bowels, and of course, in very small numbers, uteri, faces and limbs. Transplantation is far from common practice in many parts of the world, as can be seen below.

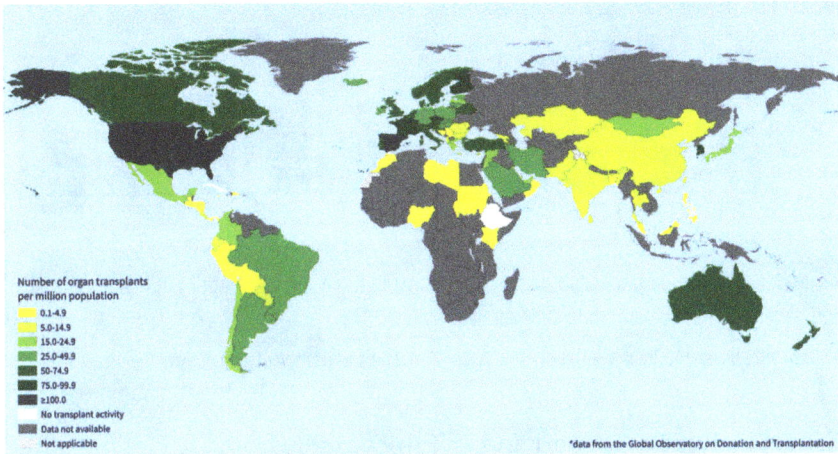

Figure 1.2. Global transplantation activities of solid organs, 2021.

Source: Data of the WHO-ONT Global Observatory on Donation and Transplantation in *International Report on Organ Donation and Transplantation Activities 2021*

Figure 1.3 hones in on the UK experience since 2013 for transplants overall. The dark blue shows the number of donors, and these always fall well below the number of patients waiting for a transplant. Unfortunately every year hundreds of patients die waiting for a life-saving organ.

So here we are, with uterine transplantation sitting at a little over 100 cases worldwide – very much at the beginning of the process. As you have already seen, our team went through a long and tortuous process, requiring sign-off from the Human Tissue Authority; a change to Oxford University Hospitals' (OUH) licence; special inspections; the approval of NHS Blood and Transplant, OUH Research and Development, and OUH Senior Management Team; Directorate and Divisional approval; and approval from NHS England. The living donor programme additionally required the approval of the Trust Advisory

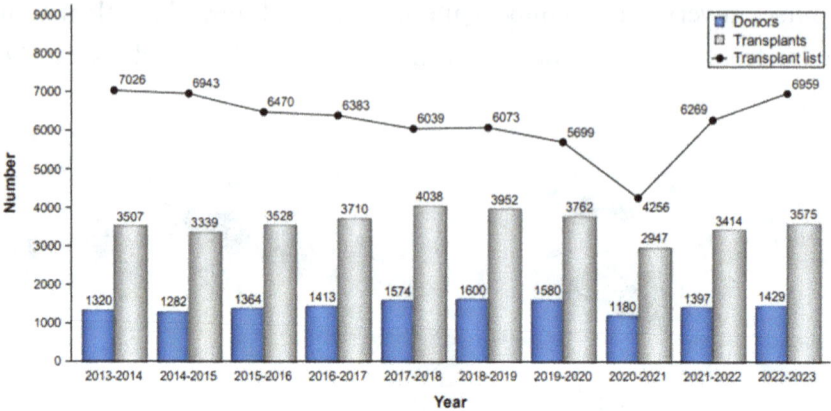

Figure 1.3. Number of deceased donors and transplants in the UK, 1 April 2013–31 March 2023, and patients on the active transplant list at 31 March 2023.

Source: NHS Blood and Transplant, *Organ and Tissue Donation and Transplantation Activity Report 2022/23*

Group, University Support and an Ethics expert from OUH. Dr Andrea Devaney and I spent many hours over five years writing and rewriting protocols in this process.

The importance of these extensive regulatory processes is absolutely validated when we look at, for example, graft survival of kidney transplant in the 1990s, which then had a 10% failure rate, primarily attributed to thrombosis in the graft's renal vein. This has now dropped to a 1% failure rate. With the early uterine transplants in living donors, there has been a 20% failure rate and a 25% failure rate in deceased donors.

International History of Womb Transplants

It has now been more than two decades since the first uterine transplant was performed in humans. The first case was performed in 2000 in Saudi Arabia using a living donor. The recipient had had her womb removed six months previously to save her life following childbirth after she had experienced excessive bleeding. Unfortunately, this transplant was unsuccessful, and the uterus needed to be removed 99 days post-implantation. This case was unquestionably undertaken prematurely; at the time we, along with Swedish and American research teams, were still undertaking essential animal-based research that would eventually provide important information to optimise the technique in humans.

More than a decade later the second uterine transplant attempt was made in Türkiye, this time using a deceased donor, and a recipient who had Mayer-Rokitansky-Küster-Hauser Syndrome (MRKH). The next nine cases were performed by Mats Brännström's team in Sweden in 2012 and 2013, using directed living donors, who were mostly the recipients' mothers.

Finally, in 2014, after decades of research, the first baby born following a uterus transplant was reported in Sweden, which demonstrated the procedure really worked. Eight live births were achieved in the cohort of nine women. The success in Sweden paved the way for the procedure to be undertaken all over the world. The first live birth using a deceased donor was achieved in Brazil in 2017. Whilst the details from a number of cases remain unpublished, our team published a review of 45 uterine transplant (or UTx) cases, which remains the most comprehensive review of the outcomes following uterus transplantation. We concluded that 10% of the living donors suffered complications that needed further surgical intervention, highlighting the potential risk involved; for example, more than a quarter of cases eventually required the transplanted uterus to be removed due to complications. In spite of these challenges, more than 100 transplants have now been performed, and more than 50 babies have been born following the procedure, highlighting without question that uterus transplantation is viable as a fertility-restoring treatment for women without a functional uterus.

2

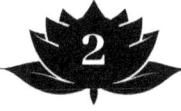

Attitudes Towards
Womb Transplants

Media Issues

Uterine transplant as a project has always stimulated strong feelings amongst colleagues, and it has engendered huge frenzies of media activity over the years.

The first time this happened I displayed great naivety. One of my junior doctors had been at a party and got into conversation with a *Sunday Times* journalist, who then phoned me up when I was in the middle of my main NHS Gynaecology clinic. I took the call and answered a few questions. The following weekend I was starting a week's holiday. That Sunday morning, I walked to the local newsagent and duly bought the paper. I got home, placed it on the kitchen table, and started looking through the general sections, but saw no sign of the piece. Then I looked at the medical section – nothing there, either. I relaxed and set about preparing my cooked breakfast (a full Scottish on a Sunday). After serving up, I sat down and turned the paper over – it was the front-page headline! At that point I thought I had better phone the hospital Press Office; they were not happy, and even less so when I told them I was off to Cornwall with no telephone contact. I ran away, which was not a bad tactic, in retrospect.

The next potential flashpoint came when we had finished our first series of transplants with very poor results. I had mentioned to David

Harrop, the CEO of the Lister Hospital at that time, that we might call a press conference. He sent along his media man, Neil Huband, to advise us. This was a memorable meeting. At Chelsea and Westminster Hospital I had a tiny office, with no windows, but attractively furnished (not by the NHS, but at my expense). I was sitting with Faris Zakaria, Fellow at the time; we were both in pinstripe suits. Neil walked in, smiled and said 'What are you boys up to, then?,' I replied, 'We are thinking of holding a press conference.' Neil looked us both up and down and said, 'Not in those bloody suits' – he had a point, even in the late 90s. I felt his lapel and said 'M&S, I reckon.' We all laughed, and Neil has been a friend ever since – for the record, there was no press conference, nor has there ever been.

A few years later after a further splurge of publicity, I walked into the Lister Hospital. The previous day I had talked to a journalist from the *Daily Mail*. At the end of the interview, I had said to her, 'You are bored by this project. You think it's boring!' Her response was pretty non-committal. Imagine my shock, then, when the interview was the whole of the front page. As soon as I saw it, I knew my day would fall apart as the frenzy built. These are very stressful days indeed, and happily they only occur about every three to five years.

Anyway, back to the Lister Hospital; I walked through to the lifts, where I met a female colleague who congratulated me on my work. One floor later, another surgical consultant stepped into the lift. He said, 'Richard, your research is total crap, what are you doing?'. Ten minutes later, I walked into the operating theatre coffee room, where a plastic surgeon said, 'Well done Richard, your research is great, keep going!' Wow, was this a project generating strong emotions!

The same thing kept happening when we applied for grants. In the Roche transplant awards, we came 271st out of 272 submissions. This led us to have Srdjan look at healthcare worker attitudes toward uterine transplantation, which we touch on later in this chapter. In conjunction with Dr Alex Clarke, Srdjan also studied the psychological aspects of those women who were now approaching us; Alex designed the psychological studies around the Royal Free Face transplant programme. Thanks to her, we were able to replicate similar methods of study for our patient group.

Over the years, there have been many surges of publicity. These, of course, culminated in the summer of 2023, when we announced our first transplant. There was an enormous amount of planning involved. The stakeholders included Imperial College, Oxford University Hospitals, HCA, the Human Tissue Authority, NHS Blood and Transplant, our Patrons, and the Womb Transplant UK charity – all parties with their own public relations teams, making for a complex equation. Happily, there was agreement between all the parties as to how to proceed, and in the main, the media response was highly positive. Richard and Isabel had given interviews to the Press Association, BBC and the *Daily Mail* prior to the announcement.

We appeared on the front page of all the national papers; we were on BBC TV from morning to evening, with Isabel and Richard landing the prime *BBC Radio 4 Today* programme slot between 7.52 and 8.00 am. We both knew that was when the Prime Minister and every Cabinet Minister was likely to be listening.

That morning had a shaft of humour. Isabel was at home in Oxford; I was at my remote family house on the Isle of Bute in the western isles of Scotland. I duly woke at 6.30, went downstairs, switched on *Radio 4* and heard Fergus Walsh, the BBC Medical Editor, being interviewed about our story.

I was feeling reasonably relaxed until I switched my computer on. There was no internet connection; it transpired that a cow had walked into an electricity pylon (a wooden pole!) at the southern end of the island and caused a power cut. I needed a code but the house had no mobile phone reception. I ran down the drive in the rain – it's about a hundred yards till you find reception – and obtained my code, which was time-limited. I ran back to the house, and glory be, I was reconnected. I sat down and entered the *Today* virtual studio, when I realised my dog had crept into the room and was lying behind me snoring! I needed to get her out of there — however, as soon as I moved her, she started barking. Then, to my horror, I remembered: my mother usually appears with *her* dog around this time, and they both bark at each other! This was all very stressful. I ran upstairs and asked my mother to stay with her dog in her bedroom till 8.00 am had passed. Meanwhile my dog had returned to the settee and started snoring again. I asked the engineer if he could hear the snoring: to my enormous relief he could not. This resolution only happened by 7.45; it's no wonder I have blood pressure issues!

The interview itself went really well, with Isabel giving an important feminine perspective to the story. During the rest of that day the story went round the world, being first up on TV across the Middle East.

In September 2023, the British Embassy in Madrid reached out to Isabel and invited her to visit them in her role as a Spanish scientist based in the UK. From this came the proposal that she should participate in the British Government programme 'Pint of Science,' which is designed to promote scientific collaboration across countries. These are meetings held across Europe in famous bars. The May 2024 event featured an English and a Scottish scientist, both working in Madrid on biomedicine, and Isabel, who was working in surgical research in the UK. The first event was held in the morning at the British Embassy in Madrid, where a famous Spanish journalist from *El Mundo* conducted a round-table discussion.

A further interview then took place with Isabel for the newspaper. The next part of the programme was held in a famous bar in Madrid where intellectuals have met for decades. It started with a podcast recorded for the Embassy by Isabel and Richard in the square outside, and then moved into the bar, which rapidly filled with supporters of the three speakers, as well as the wider public. This proved a very lively event indeed, with good science from all three speakers and much beer consumed by the observers. A lot of fun was had by all.

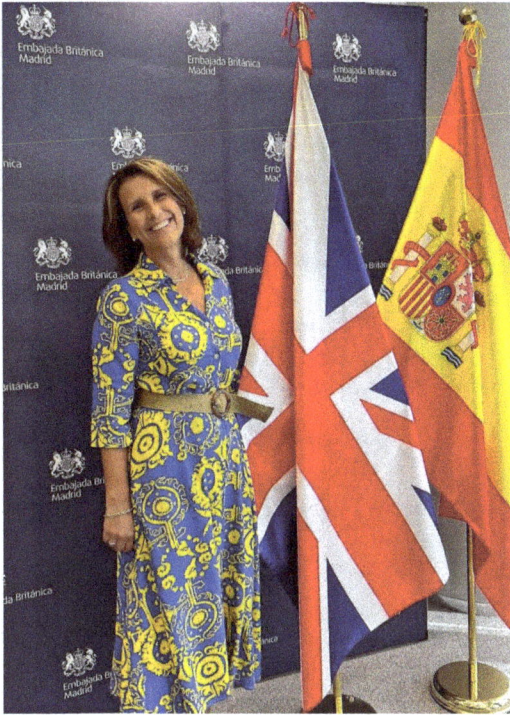

Isabel at the British Embassy in September 2023.

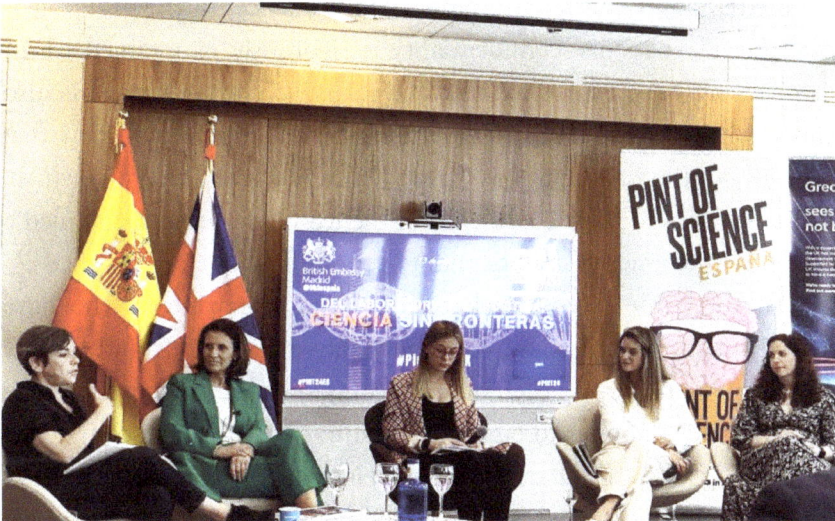

Meeting at the British Embassy, May 2024.

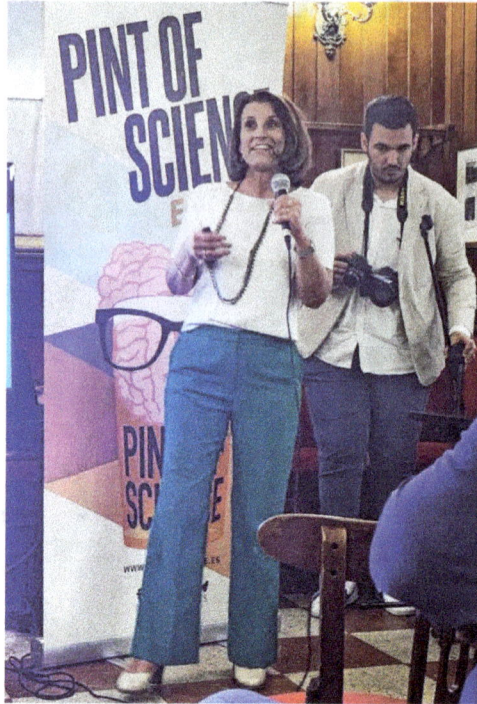

The pub-based evening 'Pint of Science' was led by Isabel, who was on excellent form.

Media issues continue to have a big influence on the group. It is vital that the patients' confidentiality is rigorously maintained whilst also sharing our progress within the scientific community. It is also important that new patients presenting to the programme know that they are not the first, and that we are building a track record — which, of course, adds to their confidence in the team. However, social media makes maintenance of confidentiality very difficult.

Another unforeseen development is that the patients who have gone through the procedure have inevitably met in clinic and formed their own bonds, giving each other ongoing support in their respective journeys. The team has to be acutely aware of the potential confidentiality pitfalls here. The charity has been blessed by having Neil Huband, an ex-BBC newsman and highly skilled public-relations guru, to look after these issues. Neil also fields all the media inquiries to the charity and has helped us walk the tightrope of not wishing to court publicity, but also being open enough to allow for fundraising and our responsibility to inform the public of our progress.

This was exemplified recently when Richard and Isabel lectured at the Royal Institution of Great Britain in London. With the exception of Albert Einstein and Stephen Hawking, no Nobel laureate in science and medicine has failed to lecture there. This is the same lecture theatre where Michael Faraday described his discovery of electricity; Sir Humphry Davy presented his invention of the Davy lamp; and Sir James Dewar, the vacuum flask. Dewar, interestingly, was a former pupil of Dollar Academy in Scotland, the same school at which Richard also studied. He clearly remembers his French teacher telling him and his classmates, 'You are all stupid. The only genius this school ever had was Dewar.' Still true to this day.

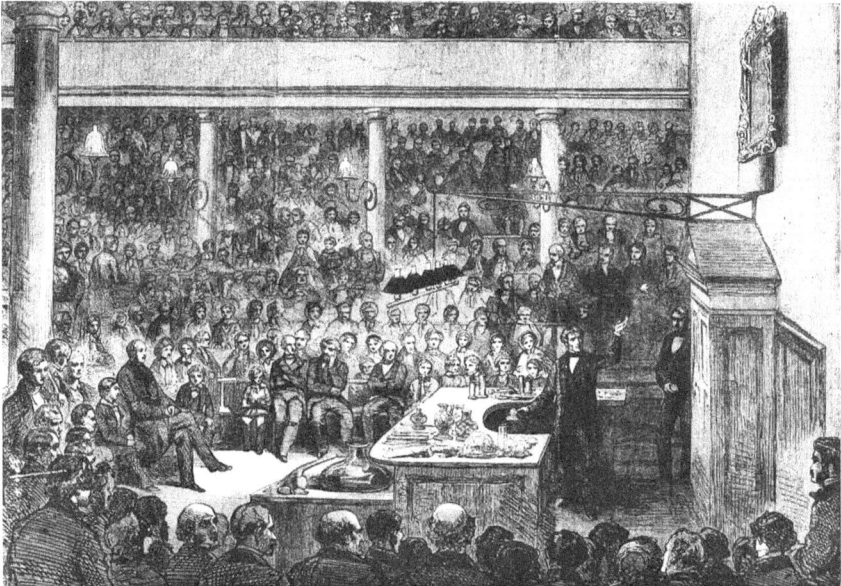

Michael Faraday presenting at the Faraday Table in the Royal Institution. The caption reads: 'Professor Faraday lecturing at the Royal Institution, before H.R.H. Price Albert, Prince of Wales, and Price Alfred — From a sketch by Alexander Blaikley.'

Source: *The Illustrated London News*, 16 February 185, v. 28, Jan–Jun. p. 177

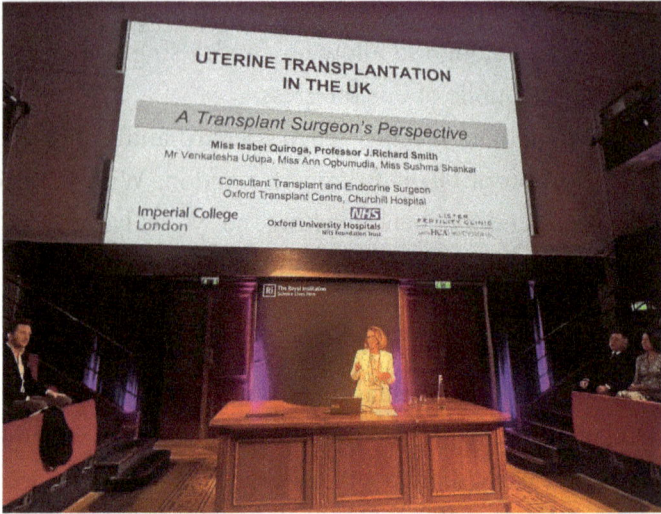

Isabel presenting at the Royal Institution. Note the Faraday table, behind which Isabel stands.

The theatre has the heavy weight of history hanging over it. It was a huge honour to be asked. Again, however, media issues were very important. There were 350 people in the theatre, but also 1,000 on livestream, and 1.5 million subscribers to the Royal Institution's YouTube channel. There was much preparation on our part and anxiety on the PR front. Happily, all went off well, with photos to prove it.

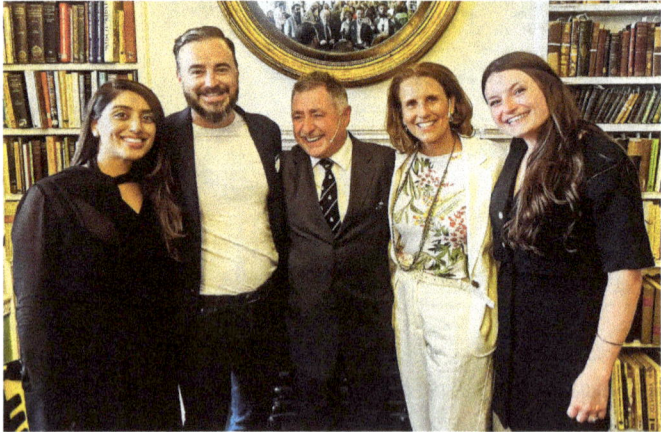

Saaliha, Ben, Richard, Isabel and Ari (left to right).

For those wishing to see this lecture, it is available via the charity website and on Youtube.[1] The whole team are very grateful to Neil, along with Piers Wright from Imperial College's PR team and Roy Probert from Oxford University Hospitals' PR team. These three individuals have certainly guided us through some stormy waters and continue to do so.

We brace for a lot more media attention when babies are born. We also know that things have the potential go wrong in any surgery or birthing situation, generating much adverse publicity. Without our PR support, this project could never have flourished.

Perspectives of Healthcare Workers[2]

We wanted to make uterine transplant more transparent and understandable to colleagues. To that end, we performed a large, in-depth survey investigating healthcare professionals' opinions on uterine transplant. The study investigated the opinions and views of UK healthcare professionals toward uterine transplant, who ranked those issues by importance.

The participants were UK transplant professionals (surgeons, nurses, operating room staff, and donor coordinators) and obstetricians and gynaecologists (trainees, members, and fellows of the Royal College of Obstetricians and Gynaecologists). The questionnaires were given out at hospital grand rounds, trainee teaching days, and conferences (both national and international). The main questions were, 'Should uterine transplant take place?' and 'Is uterine transplant achievable?'

---

[1] https://www.youtube.com/watch?v=rNFjs2Ev3q8.

[2] This section is adapted from Saso S, Clarke A, Bracewell-Milnes A, et al. Progress in Transplantation. 2015; 25: 56-63. ©2015 NATCO, The Organization for Transplant Professionals. doi: http://dx.doi.org/10.7182/pit2015552.

This article was published in 2015, but was written much earlier, before the Swedish success was published in 2014, meaning that at the time Srdjan, and thus we, had no knowledge of the Swedish programme.

In addition, we were keen to see the ranked order of importance of key issues related to uterine transplant.

The study had 528 participants at closure. An impressive 93.8% – 495 out of 528 participants – demonstrated overall support for uterine transplant as a possible future therapeutic option for absolute uterine factor infertility, with the condition that it be considered medically, surgically and ethically appropriate. Around 302 (57.2%) thought it was an achievable objective. Issues related to immunology of uterine transplant and pregnancy after uterine transplant were unanimously thought of as most important. It was also widely expressed that more effort was required to educate healthcare professionals about the procedure.

There is a two-way flow here, with any innovative and new surgical procedure bringing with it a potentially polarised ethical debate. One of the ways of moving an innovation closer to reality (i.e., the clinical setting) is by assessing and gathering support among colleagues, namely healthcare professionals. This process also allowed the uterine transplant team to gather ideas about what may need improving, or what may need to be removed from the programme, in order for it to become feasible in the future.

Published material from research related to the other recent 'life-improving' transplants (e.g., face transplants) formed the model for this needed research. Some parallels between face transplant and potential uterine transplant patients are evident, as both sets of patients are planned to undergo a transplant to improve quality of life, rather than requiring one to save their life. Furthermore, similarly to uterine transplant, face transplant is an innovative and novel procedure, and it endured a plethora of criticism and debate before being accepted by both the public and scientific body.

The UK Face team had assessed the level of support among colleagues as well as professionals who deal with transplant surgery. A high level of support for facial transplant was revealed, with 76% of respondents in favour in principle, and none opposed to it. Areas of concern highlighted in the UK Face team's study were mainly factors that affect organ retrieval, and the procedure's impact on the retrieval team and the donor family. We followed a similar path of questioning.

In this way, a large, in-depth survey investigating healthcare professionals' opinions on uterine transplant was devised. The survey consisted of a simple questionnaire that took a maximum of 15 minutes to complete, and had a format similar to the one used and validated by the face transplant team. Validation was performed by the uterine transplant research team, as well as the first 20 respondents, who assessed whether the questionnaire asked what it should about uterine transplant. Content validation was done by a focus group of transplant coordinators (London Transplant Network Coordinators), who determined that the questionnaire addressed the topic overall.

The two target populations were transplant professionals (surgeons, nurses, operating room staff, transplant and donor coordinators) and obstetricians and gynaecologists (trainees, members and fellows of the Royal College of Obstetricians and Gynaecologists [RCOG]).

While sampling the two different groups, information was gathered relating to attitudes toward practical issues of uterine retrieval and grafting; professionals' concerns for the recipient, her baby, and donor families; and the impact of these on the uterine transplant programme as a whole. The group of transplant professionals came from teaching and nonteaching hospitals in the UK, as well as from study days organised by transplant coordinators. Mainly because of geography, the London Donor Transplant Coordinators Team helped with organizing the relevant information days. As this was a gynaecological project, the biggest group was obstetricians and gynaecologists. In order to obtain a national sample distribution, members and fellows of the RCOG were sampled on a national basis.

There were opportunities to give out questionnaires to participants at hospital grand round days, trainee teaching days, and conferences (national and international). A letter explaining our project, with the questionnaire and an envelope (with our address stamped on it) attached to it, was sent out to all of the Fellows of the RCOG.

The questionnaires were designed by using closed-ended questions to allow for appropriate statistical analysis of quantitative data. The five key areas covered were:

1. general concepts related to uterine transplant (operation technique, time length, complications, immunology, achieving pregnancy after transplant, maintaining pregnancy, and risks to foetus and child development);
2. uterine retrieval and grafting (development of donor criteria, liaison with other retrieval teams, and surgical and technical issues);
3. pregnancy with a transplanted uterus (well-being of mother and foetus, and immunosuppressant effects);
4. retrieval team (education of other health professionals about uterine transplant, development of a specific patient uterine transplant team, impact of uterine transplant on operating room and intensive care unit staff, support for health professionals, negative impact on other transplant programmes, and press intrusion for health professionals and patients); and
5. donor family (likelihood of benefit for recipient, long-term support for donor family, discussion of process involved, interest in a baby from a donor family, consent issues and consent form, and press intrusion for donor family).

Participants were also asked to rank various issues related to uterine transplant, allowing each issue to be ordered according to its importance. We refer to *importance* in this case specifically with respect to uterine transplant research and future attempts at uterine transplant in humans, as well as the procedure's relative importance in comparison to other issues.

In addition to the overall results discussed above, 41.9% of respondents were adamant that more funding and grants should be made available for novel and innovative fields such as uterine transplant, instead of focusing it all on life-saving research programmes such as cancer research. About 65% indicated that they would be happy to donate their uterus to the donor registry if this option were available.

Interestingly, among transplant professionals (Transplant Surgeons and Donor Coordinators), about 54.1% (40/74) felt undecided as to whether benefits outweighed the risks of uterine transplant, with 24.3% (18/74) believing that they did, and 21.6% (16/74) stating, conversely, that the risks outweigh the benefits. Only 9.5% (7/74) thought that the development of uterine transplant would not lead to greater happiness of patients, but 44.6% were undecided (33/74). With respect to bringing benefit to medicine in general, more than 50% of respondents thought that the development of uterine transplant would also lead to a furthering of the medical, surgical, gynaecological, and transplant fields. About two-thirds of respondents (66.2%, or 49/74) thought that uterine transplant was achievable; 32.4% (24/74) were not sure; and only 4.1% (3/74) thought that uterine transplant should never take place. About 39.2% (29/74) believed that uterine transplant procedures should become available 'as soon as possible.'

Amongst the obstetricians and gynaecologists (Trainees, Members, and Fellows of the RCOG), 47.4% (136/287) thought that the benefits of uterine transplant outweighed the risks, 37.3% (107/287) were undecided, and only 15.3% (44/287) stated that the risks of uterine transplant outweighed the benefits. About 14.3% (41/287) thought that development of uterine transplant would not lead to greater happiness of patients, but 31.7% were undecided (91/287). Therefore, the majority (54%) believed that clinical uterine transplant would lead to greater human happiness. More than 60% of these respondents also thought that the development of uterine transplant would also lead to a furthering of the medical, surgical, and transplant fields more broadly. A total of 68.6% (197/287) of this group thought that uterine transplant was achievable, 27.2% (78/287) were not sure, and only 8.4% (24/287) thought that uterine transplant should never take place. Almost half (47.7%, or 137/287) believed that uterine transplant should become available as soon as possible.

The Fellows of the Royal College of Obstetricians and Gynaecology were more reserved about the procedure; of the most senior members, only 23.1% (30/130) thought that the benefits of uterine transplant outweighed the risks, 54.6% (71/130) were undecided, and 22.3% (29/130) stated that the risks of uterine transplant outweighed the benefits. About 24.6% (32/130) thought that the development of uterine transplant would not lead to greater happiness of patients, but 42.3% were undecided (55/130). 33.1% (43/130) stated that clinical uterine transplant would lead to greater human happiness. With respect to bringing benefit to medicine in general, less than 22% of respondents thought that the development of uterine transplant would not lead to a furthering of the medical, surgical, gynaecological, and transplant fields. A total of 54.6% (71/130) thought that uterine transplant was achievable, 40.8% (53/130) were not sure, and 12.3% (16/130) thought that it should never take place. About 38.5% (50/130) believed that uterine transplant should become available as soon as possible. This was pretty much as one might expect, as seniority often leads to conservatism.

We also looked at respondents who had encountered personal issues with infertility; unsurprisingly, this group were in general the most supportive.

The levels of importance of specific individual issues with respect to achieving a successful uterine transplant were also ranked. Issue groups 1 through 5 consisted of issues specific to uterine transplant; procedural issues; retrieval issues; recipient issues; and donor issues. These were ranked according to how important they were considered in bringing about a successful uterine transplant procedure and, subsequently, a healthy child. The ranking was both overall and according to profession. Issues related to immunology of uterine transplant and pregnancy after uterine transplant were unanimously thought of as most important. Ranked second were recipient-related issues, which overlapped significantly with the issues in the first group (e.g., pregnancy, immunosuppressants, and risks to foetus). Issues related to organ harvest were ranked third. Donor and procedure-related issues were ranked at the bottom. Participants' sex and profession did not seem to affect their ranking of uterine transplant issues.

The research concluded that uterine transplant appeared to be supported by healthcare professionals in the UK, with 94% wanting its clinical application, provided that all the criteria were met, and 57% stating that they thought it achievable. Therefore, we could conclude that there was no majority objection to uterine transplant in principle.

Generally, it seemed that the healthcare profession was supportive of uterine transplant as an idea to restore fertility, but a significant proportion, 40% to 50%, were not confident that uterine transplant would ever get to a clinical stage. Three reasons may explain that hesitance: (1) belief that the risks of uterine transplant to both the mother and foetus are significant enough to prevent uterine transplant in humans; (2) conviction that transplant and non-rejection of a uterine graft may be possible, yet the graft will not able to carry a term pregnancy; and (3) the new procedure's financial implications for an already cash-strapped National Health Service.

When analysing the results according to the sub-groups, no real difference was seen between the percentages when compared with the overall results discussed above. The results were a strong indication that research on uterine transplant, and the present direction of UK human uterine transplant attempt was heading toward had a strong base of support among colleagues.

The third group surveyed, which included the more senior and experienced obstetricians and gynaecologists, were also supportive overall, but definitely more cautious. There was a noticeably smaller proportion of those fellows who thought that uterine transplant was achievable, at 54.6% in comparison to 66–68% recorded from the first two groups surveyed. Also, 12.3% thought that uterine transplant should never take place – still a small proportion, but definitely higher than what was recorded for the first two groups. The seniority of the group of RCOG fellows meant that the participants were more experienced and more knowledgeable, yet also more conservative, set in their own practice and perhaps less likely to consider novel and innovative ideas.

Finally, by contrast to the group of RCOG fellows who were less supportive, the last group (participants who had experienced infertility either personally or as a couple) were more supportive than the general population and the first two groups. They had individually felt the effects of infertility on their lives, as well as their relationships. For this reason, they would be more empathic and understanding toward women who were experiencing a problem with their fertility — in this case, a type of infertility caused by a uterine factor. Importantly, those familiar with the problems that people with infertility encounter may find it easier to justify a radical and novel procedure.

This research was important and illuminating at the time. Returning to 2015, it becomes evident that the multitude of views Richard encountered on a single walk through the Lister Hospital were probably quite representative of the wider healthcare community.

Among Srdjan's other projects was a study of psychological issues in women with absolute uterine factor infertility that was published in 2016. Forty women who had presented themselves to the programme were shown an educational video prepared by the team, went through a question-and-answer session, and then were interviewed in depth. Thirty-nine (97.5%) said they would prefer undergoing uterine transplantation over surrogacy or adoption. This was despite their full knowledge that those two options were safer for the women themselves, and that the graft might fail prior to embryo transfer. All of the women felt the procedure should be available, and the vast majority thought it likely to be successful. Although this study was published after Brännström's success, the interviews were undertaken long before that success was known by any outside of the Swedish team.

• Part II •
Early Days of Fertility Preservation and Restoration

Chapter

3

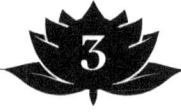

Early Explorations

The Society of Gynaecological Oncologists, 1995

In the spring of 1995, while living in New York on a sabbatical, I had the good fortune to attend the Annual Meeting of the Society of Gynaecological Oncologists (SGO) of North America, which that year was held in New Orleans. I had become friends with Giuseppe Del Priore, a New York gynaecological cancer surgeon. Giuseppe and I travelled to New Orleans and sat through many sessions together. On one morning there was an interactive teaching session, in which a very talented compère would present a slide with a medical scenario and the audience would vote on four possible answers via a device. The percentage of each vote was then displayed, and the four judges, all of whom were famous in our field, would walk us through the correct answer or answers. Most of the audience, as you would expect, usually got it right, but there were always a few outliers, to whom the judges would opine 'you know who you are, you would fail your board exams,' – cue much laughter. This was a really electric postgraduate education, with about 500 people in the audience.

Partway through this session, the judges began discussing how many vessels were needed for a uterus to be viable. As shown in Figure 3.1, there are six vessels supplying the uterus; two uterine arteries; two ovarian vessels; and two vessels supplying the vagina.

These give a collateral supply to the uterus, meaning the blood flow continues on to nearby organs. The figure also shows the ureters – the tubes that run between the kidneys and the bladder, under the uterine arteries. A classic mnemonic for generations of trainee gynaecologists has been 'the water runs under the bridge.'

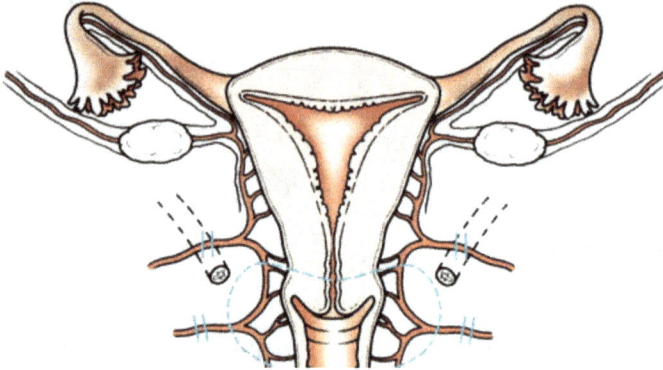

Figure 3.1. Vascular supply of the genital tract.

The first question asked whether the uterus remained viable with one vessel tied off. All of the audience correctly agreed. Next, it was asked whether the same was true if both uterine vessels were tied off. The majority still thought so. The following question asked whether the uterus would be viable should both uterine vessels, plus one ovarian vessel, be tied off. At this stage, the vast majority believed it would not. The conclusion drawn was that four of the six supplying vessels were required; the significance of this will become apparent soon.

Later that day, Giuseppe and I attended a session where the great French surgeon, Daniel Dargent (now deceased), presented his initial data on a procedure he had invented: the radical vaginal trachelectomy. At the time, he was the first doctor to remove a cervical cancer, along with its surrounding tissue (known as the parametrium), while leaving the patient with a functioning uterus. Of particular interest to us, Dargent removed the cancerous lymph nodes from the pelvis laparo-scopically. Although this is standard practice today, at the time it was revolutionary. In addition, following Dargent's procedure, the 'water runs under the bridge' no longer. Doing the procedure vaginally brings the ureter downwards. This creates what Dargent called '*le genou*' because the ureter becomes like a flexed knee, and thus much easier to accidentally damage.

Dargent had approached the ureters from below as he came up the vagina, meaning that he avoided affecting the uterine arteries; in other words, he only took out the two vaginal collaterals of the six vessels supplying the uterus. As Giuseppe and I listened to Dargent's presentation, we both agreed as to the brilliance of the idea, but we questioned whether the procedure might not be more easily done abdominally. Our issue was that if we were to do what would later be called an abdominal radical trachelectomy (ART), we would have to transect (divide) the uterine arteries to allow for full dissection of the ureters, which is the standard approach when removing a cervical cancer. In fact, at the end of a radical hysterectomy the ureters are hanging free by their insertion into the bladder. This, however, has been achieved by dividing the uterine arteries.

To digress here, traditionally, prior to Dargent's laparoscopic ('keyhole') approach, there had been four ways to remove the uterus. First, one could do a total hysterectomy, via the abdomen, involving removal of the uterus and cervix with or without the tubes and ovaries. Second, one could perform a sub-total hysterectomy, whereby the cervix is left *in situ*, or, third, a radical hysterectomy, whereby the uterus, cervix and surrounding parametrium are removed. This approach was originally described by the Viennese surgeon Wertheim at the turn of the 19th century in order to remove cancers of the cervix, and it is a longer and much more complex operation than a total hysterectomy. Fourth, surgeons could remove the uterus via the vagina, with no cuts in the abdomen; this is known as a vaginal hysterectomy. This usually is done for benign conditions and often combined with a vaginal repair-type procedure if there is laxity or prolapse.

In the 19th century, the Celia Schauta procedure, also known as the Schauta-Amreich procedure, put forth a very technically challenging radical procedure for cervical cancer that was performed via the vagina. It was then discovered that removing the cancer also required the removal of related lymph nodes, consigning the procedure to the history books for 70 years. However, the advent of the laparoscope brought the operation back to the table, in the hands of Daniel Dargent, Denis Querleu, Michel Roy and Marie Plante, four French surgeons. They showed that cervical cancer could be managed by laparoscopic removal of the nodes, followed by the Schauta radical vaginal hysterectomy. Dargent made the huge leap in realising that he could remove the cervix and parametrium and leave the uterus *in situ,* thus allowing the woman to potentially have a baby in the future.

It is important that I clarify the difference between the radical approach to the cervix and the simple benign approach, as the two operations are completely different in their technique, scope and risks. In benign gynaecological surgery, one moves carefully down the side of the uterus, keeping as far away as one can from the pelvic sidewall organs. These organs include the 'great vessels' (the common, internal, and external iliac vessels) and the nerves supplying the pelvis and the legs, as well as the ureters on the pelvic sidewall. Damage to these structures can be catastrophic and lead to lifelong debility. In the radical procedure, all of these structures are dissected out and avoided by knowing exactly where they are. All gynaecological cancer surgeons are familiar with procedures performed abdominally, but not necessarily with making this dissection via the vagina, in which the ureters, bladder, and, to a lesser extent, the bowel are all vulnerable to injury. This risk was reflected in the Dargent initial series, where up to 20% of surgeries led to the development of fistulas.[3]

---

[3] Fistulas are where a hole develops post-operatively between the urinary or intestinal tracts and the vagina, rendering the woman incontinent until the fistula is repaired — also a challenging surgery.

The Ovarian Vessel Discovery

With all of this in mind at the SGO conference in New Orleans, the dilemma remained for Giuseppe and I: our proposed approach would leave the uterus supplied by only two vessels, the ovarian vessels. How were we, then, to either preserve the uterine arteries or put them back together? As the interactive teaching class had shown earlier in the day, we did not believe that two vessels were adequate.

Later that day we took a trolley car ride through New Orleans, excitedly discussing all of this as we watched the grand Southern mansions slide by. The trolley car then slid past some less salubrious parts of New Orleans, arriving in a very downtrodden area. Giuseppe and I were in suits, shirts and ties and were no longer blending in. To our horror, the driver announced, 'everybody get off.' It was Mardi Gras, and instead of the trolley car going back down the track into the centre, we were stuck in the back of beyond. We duly disembarked, and Giuseppe asked somebody how to get back into town. He said 'You take this bus to here, and then change buses and take this bus to here, and then one more change and you will be back.' Like an idiot, I said, 'It would be easier to just take a taxi!'. Big mistake. The man then shouts 'Are you guys rich? Hey everybody, these guys are rich!' Giuseppe is then hastily shouting 'We aren't rich.' Trouble was, we looked it. I reassured the man that I was not rich but a Scottish tourist and between the two of us, we escaped by bus.

Returning to New York a few days later, Guiseppe and I sought to try our method on a formalin-preserved human cadaver at Bellevue Hospital. Here I made the unfortunate mistake of not realising that the gurney had a drainage hole; I lost a good pair of trousers and boxers that day! This sort of work is a bit gruesome, but it is essential: we discovered that we could do an abdominal trachelectomy — at least in a cadaver. Giuseppe and I have remained friends and collaborators ever since.

A few weeks later, I returned to London to the Chelsea and Westminster Hospital. On my return I applied for, and received, ethics approval to perform an ART in a woman who was already having a radical hysterectomy. At this time, we still felt as though we had no choice but to divide the uterine arteries, which we then (with the assistance of microvascular surgeons) had worked out how to suture back together, but we did prove that the tumour clearance with the radical trachelectomy was the same as with a radical hysterectomy.

However, we were left with yet another problem. Imagine that you have an accident resulting in your hand being cut off; when the microvascular surgeons stitch it back on, they will use very fine sutures to repair the vessels. The newly restored (anastomosed) vessels will function normally, but the suturing means that they will remain the same diameter for the rest of your life. This is not a problem for most vessels, but the case is different for uterine vessels. The uterus, in its non-pregnant state, is the size of a pear, and its uterine arteries are two to three millimetres in diameter. At full term, the pregnant uterus is the size of a watermelon and the uterine arteries are 10 millimetres in diameter. We therefore were worried that the suture line would create an hourglass effect during pregnancy.

To address this concern, we undertook animal research with help from the wonderful Professor David Noakes, formerly Vice Principal of the Royal Veterinary College and Professor of Reproductive Medicine.[4] We sat the appropriate four exams and obtained ethics committee approval from the RVC, as well as the appropriate Home Office licenses, which would allow us to do a research project in a porcine model. We ultimately studied three pigs, who were cared for to the highest standards. Two had their uterine vessels divided and sutured, and in one the vessels were left intact. The animals recovered from the procedure and were mated, and all three went on to carry their piglets to term, and the piglets grew normally. We were concerned that if the blood supply was deficient, then the piglets might be growth-restricted – they weren't.

---

[4] David has supported the projects that follow over a 20-year period, and it has been a great honour and privilege to work with him and his colleagues at the RVC.

We worried that the vessels might blow out, causing massive haemorrhage – they didn't. The scans during pregnancy showed the uterine arteries functioning normally, and at the post-mortem dissection, the vessels were essentially normal and showed only minimal buildup of tissue in the arteries (intimal fibrosis).

The story now gets more complicated. At that time, we (David Corless, Faris Zakaria and I) were working at the Royal Veterinary College (RVC) on the project described above, and we had also presented our preliminary case at the British Gynaecological Cancer Society (BGCS). The Society had showed little interest, except for László Ungár, a Hungarian gynaecological cancer surgeon. Our teams dined together, and we agreed to collaborate. Some of our people, including Dr Deborah Boyle, went to Budapest to assist László in the first ART that did not lead to the patient losing her uterus. Although László had arranged for a microvascular surgeon to be in attendance, after the ART was complete, the uterus looked completely pink and viable without its uterine arteries. This was the key to much that followed: the uterus, cervix, and ovaries *could* all be supported by the two ovarian vessels alone (see Figure 3.2).

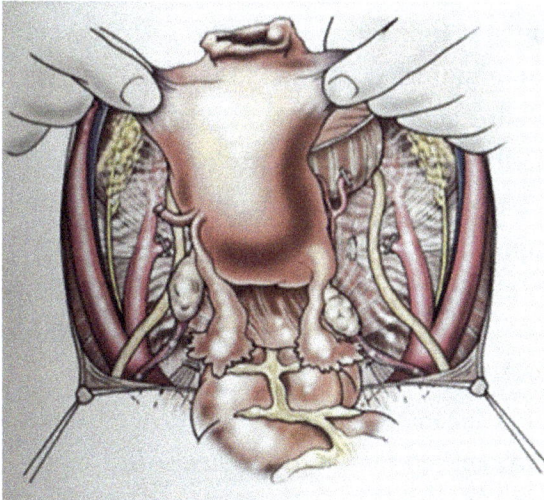

Figure 3.2. The uterus outside the abdomen connected via the ovarian blood vessels.

Despite this massive leap forward, at this point none of us knew whether anastomosed (surgically connected) vessels would work: we were only mid-way through this work at the RVC, and were still concerned about the hourglass effect or, even worse, a blow-out and haemorrhage during pregnancy. László had dispensed with the re-suturing of the uterine vessels, and instead replaced the body of the uterus (minus its cervical cancer) into the abdomen by suturing it on at the vagina. László rapidly built a series of cases; no longer bound by our worries that four vessels were needed to support the uterus, Giuseppe and I followed.

We then sought to understand why the ovarian vessels alone were adequate to supply not just the ovaries, but also the uterus. We performed a number of human cadaveric dissections at the human anatomy department at Charing Cross Hospital. We discovered that the structure known as the ovarian ligament was no 'ligament.' It in fact contains three vessels: one artery, and two veins. The ovarian artery runs down directly from the aorta to the ovary, where it divides, giving a blood supply to the ovary. A branch then tracks round the ovary into the 'ligament,' thus supplying the uterus. Two veins take the opposite course from the uterus round the ovary, coalescing into the ovarian veins higher up and thus returning to the Inferior Vena Cava (IVC). Our research and findings occurred in the mid 90s as part of Deborah Boyle's research, in conjunction with histopathologist Dr Ian Lindsay.

This then led on to a project where we looked at blood supply to the uterus, measuring it by measuring uterine perfusion as the blood supply was sequentially cut off during a routine hysterectomy. This work formed the basis of Paul Moxey's BSc and was a small part of Krishen Sieunarine's PhD thesis. This project is described in Chapter 4 covering spin-off discoveries.

Our research meant that we now understood a little better why two vessels were able to do the trick. It also led to the observation that, when outside the abdomen during the procedure, the uterus was almost detached from the body, with the exception of the two vessels that we had identified. In performing the procedure, the surgeon literally brings the uterus, cervix, parametrium, and transected upper vagina out of the abdomen. The surgeon then cuts off the cervix (with the cancer), parametrium, and upper vagina before re-suturing the remaining uterus and thin cervical plate back onto the vagina.

Our porcine experiment also meant we were confident the arteries could be anastomosed and thus function in pregnancy. As it was now obvious that uterine arterial anastomosis was not required as part of ART, it led the way to uterine transplant becoming a real possibility.

With this knowledge, my first stop was to arrange to go for a drink with Mr Sam Abdalla, Director of Lister Fertility Clinic, which was at that time the UK's largest free-standing fertility clinic. Sam is an internationally famous infertility expert. Sam and I had worked together since 1983 when we first met in Glasgow. He confirmed that this technique could help many women who could not conceive because of absolute uterine factor infertility. This conversation led us to return to the RVC, where we obtained Ethics and Home Office's permission to auto-transplant eight pigs. With Krishen as our Fellow, we took our subjects to theatre, removed the uterus, and carefully preserved the uterine arteries and veins. These were then skilfully sutured by surgeon and friend, Mr David Corless. The immediate results were impressive, but total failure ensued in the longer term. There was extensive microvascular thrombosis – in other words, clots formed in the small vessels, making the uterus shrink to such a small size as to be unworkable.

Early Attempts at Uterine Transplants in the 2000s

It was the year 2000, and the porcine series had produced some amazing spin off projects: the law of unintended consequences was hard at work. (Some of these will be expanded upon in the following chapter.) However, we were no closer to being able to successfully transplant a uterus.

In 2002, Dr Wafa'a Fageeh's team, from Saudi Arabia, published the first attempt at uterine transplantation in a woman that they had performed in 2000, having run a set of animal-based experiments that was similar ours. Sadly, the transplant failed after three months and had to be removed. The human uterus developed microvascular thrombosis – blood clots – just as we had found with our pigs. I really thought the project was over. Before giving up, though, I knew that I should chew the issue over with a transplant surgeon.

I visited Professor Nadey Hakim at St Mary's Hospital, which is part of Imperial College. Nadey has been a supporter of this project ever since, for which I am forever grateful. At the time, however, he simply told me that we were 'doing it wrong': instead of suturing small vessels, we needed to utilise a large vessel patch technique. This involved retrieval of the much bigger vessels on the pelvic sidewall and possibly the aorta and IVC. This technique was being used in pancreas and small-bowel transplants, which were being pioneered at the time.

Our team duly practiced this dissection on a formalin-preserved human cadaver at Charing Cross Hospital, and then on a fresh cadaveric pig at the RVC. The results were amazing: the graft incorporated the aorta, IVC, common and internal iliac arteries and veins,

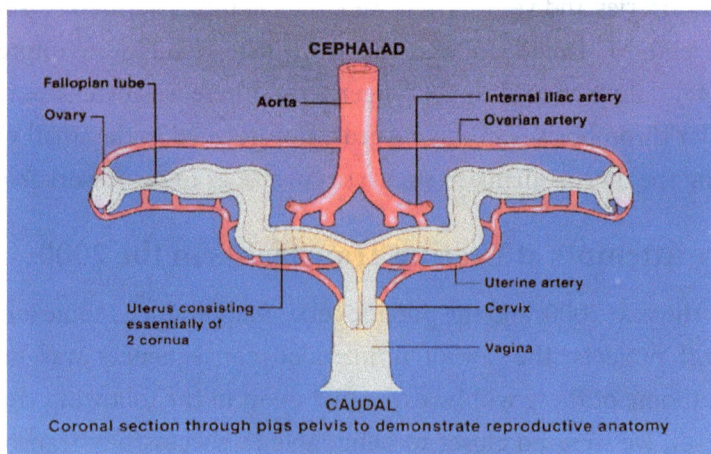

Figure 3.3. The anatomy in both the pig and rabbit (although note that these are of very different sizes), with a single cervix and vagina connected to two long horns of the uterus; note that these are of very different sizes. The vascular anatomy is quite similar to that of a woman.

along with the uterine arterio-venous tree, and, of course, the uterus, cervix, and upper vagina (see Figure 3.3).

The success of the technique became evident when we cannulated the aorta and poured fluid through the graft — and there was no leakage. The blood started to flow out of the IVC, and then out flowed the clear fluid that we were pouring in. Within five minutes the uterus had gone from being pink in colour to pure white. Here we finally had a graft that might work! It might seem obvious now, but until that point, I had never clocked that the pelvic organs are pink because of the blood within them.

Professor Noakes at the RVC undertook a small mountain of paperwork to secure permissions to run a series of transplants to be performed in rabbits from one animal to another — up to this point, we had only undertaken an auto-transplant, in which we removed and then replaced the same uterus into the pig. Professor Noakes and Dr Michael Boyd provided the veterinary care. Krishen remained the Fellow for our first series, in which we had brilliant immediate intra-operative results, but more disappointing long-term results. Although we learnt much from that first series of six transplants, a number of rabbits sadly died of pulmonary embolism. Dr Anna David, Consultant Obstetrician at University College, London, joined the project as an advisor when she realised and pointed out to us that we were not performing ultrasound on our subjects, and we started doing so. Concurrently with this, Krishen and Ian Lindsay looked at tissue viability in 12 cold-stored human uteruses. From this we concluded that the uterus was definitely good for 12 hours outside of the body, and probably good for 24 hours.

At this point, our high rate of pulmonary embolism became our biggest worry. If in trouble — call a friend! Over dinner, Nadey Hakim and I discussed the team's intra-operative approach, assisted by many hand gestures. When I described our technique for the retrieval and the perfusion of the graft, I began miming compressing a syringe. Nadey picked up on this immediately: 'What's that?' he asked as he emulated the syringe action. I explained that we perfused the uterus using a syringe and canula into the aorta. This, Nadey thought, was the root of our troubles: our syringe was blowing lacunae (islands) into the graft, which then formed clots. Instead, he suggested, we should perfuse with a glass bottle, which would ensure that no pressure could be applied. This put us right on our organ perfusion technique. Patience is of the essence here; when the perfusion starts with gravity as the only feed, the process is very slow, with just little drips of fluid at first, before it naturally becomes a flow. Nadey also commented that this mistake had been made in the early days of organ transplant with kidneys.

On the back of this advice, our next series proved much more successful. Two animals were mated to achieve a potential pregnancy, but were unable to conceive. We euthanised one of the two long-term survivors and discovered a tubal blockage. We thereafter applied for permission to perform IVF to allow embryo transfer, but unfortunately, the week that we obtained permission, the surviving animal developed severe diarrhoea and sadly demised. This was all happening throughout the early 2000s.

In 2010, Srdjan Saso became the team's new Fellow, and he set about multiple projects, including arranging IVF for our animals. We later succeeded in inducing a pregnancy with embryos brought from Valencia and Prof Jimenez's laboratory. This was a great achievement, being only the third case in the world where pregnancy had been achieved in a fully transplanted uterus. We had also started collaborating with Neil Clancy, a biophotonic physicist who had a novel method of looking at uterine blood flow — an optical densitometry technique — which has proved a useful adjunct to the perfusion index and pulse oximetry. We will touch on this in more detail when discussing fertility-sparing surgery (see page 49).

Chapter

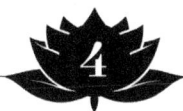

Spin-Off Projects

Before we continue with the uterine transplant journey, we are going to take some time out to explore new procedures we have developed to allow women with certain cancers to have fertility-sparing surgery, as recounted by Richard. Historically, management of gynaecological cancers has often resulted in infertility because the uterus and/or ovaries needed to be removed. As our research into uterine transplant involved a much greater understanding of the blood supply to and from the uterus, so new procedures were developed for cancer patients.

Abdominal Radical Trachelectomy

You will remember that on my return from the Society of Gynaecological Oncologists in New Orleans, Guiseppe and I performed an operation that proved that the tumour clearance with the radical trachelectomy was the same as with a radical hysterectomy.

We also demonstrated that ART could be performed in early pregnancy, and that the patient could carry her baby to term. However, for ART performed during early pregnancy, the uterine arteries must be preserved: if they are transected, the patient will miscarry. In our series of five cases undertaken during early pregnancy, two women delivered healthy babies. When we perform ART in a non-pregnant patient, we advise her to wait a year until she tries for a baby, because it allows time for the ovarian vessels and vaginal collaterals to enlarge to replace the defunct uterine arteries.

More recently Alan Farthing CVO, friend, colleague, Chief of Service at the West London Gynaecological Cancer Centre and also HM the late Queen's gynaecologist, performed the world's first laparoscopic ART during pregnancy, with a successful outcome for both mother and baby. An alternative approach is to use chemotherapy. This has been used to some effect to treat cervical cancer during pregnancy. When counselling a woman in the terrible position of being diagnosed with cervical cancer during pregnancy, both approaches should be discussed. I know which one I would choose, but I also know that I am biased in this regard!

To achieve fertility-sparing surgery, the abdominal radical trachelectomy (ART) approach pioneered by our team,[5] or the laparoscopic method combined with a radical vaginal procedure, are now the order of the day for tackling cervix cancer. This has not always been the case. The consensus among surgeons is always in flux. There was a time when tumours smaller than 2 cm were operated on via the vaginal route, and larger tumours (2–4 cm) by the abdominal approach, and that was either open, laparoscopically or robotically. However, best practise changed in 2021 with the publication of a large North American series of cases of radical hysterectomy and trachelectomy performed laparoscopically or robotically. Unfortunately, the long-term follow-up with this approach showed higher recurrence rates of cervical cancer than the earlier method, and so began the sea change of opinion in favour of the open radical hysterectomy or ART.

Giuseppe, László and I can justly claim to have invented the ART operation, but in truth we reinvented it. It transpired that in Bucharest in 1932, a surgeon named Eugen Aburel had performed the same operation in four cases, and published his findings in an obscure Romanian

---

[5] The radical abdominal hysterectomy (RAH) and the laparoscopic removal of lymph nodes, combined with a vaginal approach, are also currently favoured approaches.

journal. No pregnancies were recorded. I should add that none of us had any knowledge of this publication until years after our original cases. It is every surgeon's dream to invent a procedure, and I don't think that we are any different. However, we each initially faced backlash for our approach, requiring all three of us to change jobs. Although we had proved that the tumour clearance with the radical trachelectomy was the same as with a radical hysterectomy, we endured 10 years of criticism, getting told that we didn't understand cancer, before the operation took off round the world. It was at the SGO in Palm Springs in 2007 where we finally found acceptance. I knew that the procedure was fully established when one day, while eating breakfast with my two older children, Cameron and Victoria, in a New York diner, an advert came on the radio directed at young women with cancer of the cervix, telling them 'You don't need to lose your fertility, come to Memorial Sloane-Kettering for an abdominal radical trachelectomy.' I turned to my children and said, 'That is Dad's, Giuseppe's and László's op!'.

A last point on the ART: you may have noted that we − that is, myself, Del Priore, and Ungár, − forbore from attaching our names to the procedure. Ironically, avoiding attaching our names to the procedure has allowed the French to dub it the Aburel procedure. We deliberately chose not to call it the Radical Abdominal Trachelectomy, which would of course have had the acronym RAT − not nearly as elegant as ART.

Fertility-Sparing Surgery

As alluded to on page 42, Krishen Sieunarine and medical student Paul Moxey followed Deborah Boyle's work on the ovarian ligament and the discovery, via the ART procedure, that two vessels could support the uterus. They developed a device to measure perfusion index and pulse oximetry in the porcine uterine transplant series. This was a novel idea that originated with anaesthetist, ethicist and chronic pain specialist Dr Andrew Lawson. He suggested that the probe that is placed on the patient's finger during anaesthesia could be increased in size, allowing it to be placed round the transplanted uterus.[6] Paul, now a vascular surgeon, did his BSc project on pulse oximetry and perfusion index measurement in the porcine uterine transplant series. Paul showed that this device was successful in determining uterine blood flow. This was generously supported, in equipment terms, by Datex-Ohmeda.

Although, as described earlier, our porcine transplants had failed in the long term, our research on those cases led directly to this advance in pulse oximetery. With this, we were able to move to the human setting in 2006. Krishen, Paul and I measured the blood supply to the uterus as we performed hysterectomies and selectively ligated the six supplying vessels to the uterus. Using the device, we were able to show that 40% of the supply came from the ovarian vessels, 10% from the vaginal collaterals and 50% from the uterine vessels. It allowed us to see that we could control the blood supply to the uterus during surgery, thus allowing us, with virtually no blood loss, to cut the uterus in half. We termed this the modified Strassman procedure (MSP). We realised that the standard practise of tying a rubber tube round the base of the uterus only partly worked because a large amount of the blood supply was via the ovarian vessels. However, if we dissected the individual vessels and placed vascular occlusion clips across the vessels, we could massively reduce blood loss.

Figure 4.1 shows the arteries supplying the uterus, in particular the ovarian, uterine and vaginal collateral vessels. The area in dotted blue shows the area encompassing the cervix and vagina, as well as the parametrium, which must be removed in ART.

In the MSP, bulldog clips are placed across the ovarian vessels and the uterine vessels are temporarily occluded using rubber tubing in the traditional method. Vascular bulldog clips (see Figure 4.2) — notwithstanding their weak appearance — are temporarily applied to

---

[6] Andrew was a wonderful man who sadly died after battling mesothelioma for six years. He, and many other doctors, sadly developed the rare and usually rapidly fatal condition of mesothelioma because of the asbestos in the ceiling of the medical students' accommodation at Guy's Hospital. Andrew directed his own treatment path to great success, and saw his three lovely children all become adults.

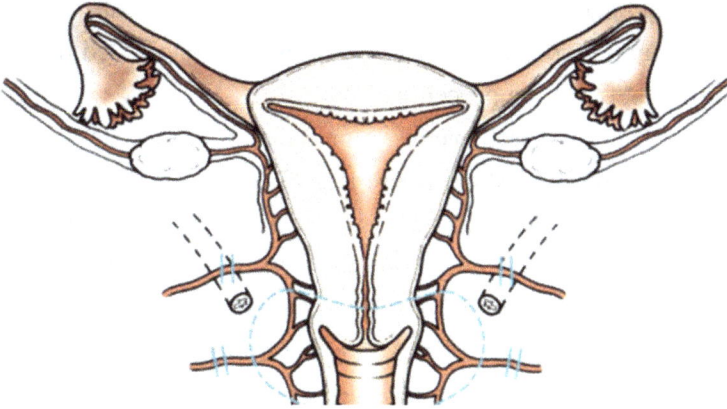

Figure 4.1. Vascular supply of the genital tract.

block to the ovarian ligaments and to the uterine arteries. The uterus can then be opened and single-site tumours removed. The first case we described was one in which the patient had a rare benign giant adenomatoid tumour of the uterus. This was removed and the uterus

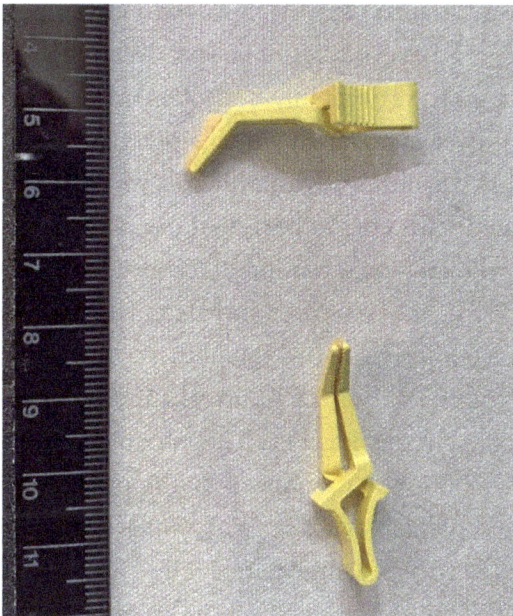

Figure 4.2. Bulldog clips.

reconstructed successfully. It is really important to point out that the porcine animal work described in the previous chapter led directly to the modified Strassman procedure.

I have had the great privilege for 30 years to be the surgeon to the National Trophoblastic Disease and Ovarian Germ Cell (tumour) Centre at Charing Cross Hospital in London. My friend and colleague Professor Michael Seckl is a world-renowned expert on this subject. Trophoblastic disease is where the placenta develops abnormally. The most benign variant of this a hydatidiform mole. In a normal pregnancy, genetic content comes from the mother via the ovum (egg) and from the father via the sperm. In gestational trophoblastic disease, the genetic content comes wholly or partially from the father. Instead of a foetus developing, the uterus fills with grape-like vesicles (the mole) – it looks a bit like frog spawn. In a complete mole, the genes are all from the father and there is no foetus. In a partial mole there is a foetus (non-viable), an abnormal placenta, and a mix of the mother and father's genes. Additionally, there is a spectrum ranging from invasive mole, to choriocarcinoma, to placental site and embryonic trophoblastic tumours (PSTTs and ETTs, respectively). Choriocarcinomas are cancers that grow very rapidly and often metastasise (spread), to the lungs, brain, liver etc. Happily, molar pregnancies and choriocarcinoma are highly chemosensitive and have a very high cure rate. They are usually treated with chemotherapy alone following evacuation of the uterus, thus allowing preservation of fertility.

PSTTs and ETTs are even rarer and also metastasise, readily. They are, however, much less sensitive to chemotherapy, and therefore harder to treat. Apart from PSTT and ETTs, all other gestational trophoblastic disease (GTD) puts out the hormone beta human chorionic gonadotrophin (beta HCG, a hormone produced by the placenta in pregnancy). This is the basis of pregnancy testing kits, which measure beta HCG in urine. Beta HCG is also measurable in blood – in fact, more accurately than in urine. With moles, the beta HCG levels can be very high; instead of 1,000 to 10,000, they can reach levels greater than 100,000, even into the millions. Very counterintuitively, patients with very high levels in their blood can have a negative urinary pregnancy test. This is down to different subunits of beta HCG. The negative urine test can lead to late diagnosis unless people remember to do a blood level test of beta HCG. The monitoring of beta HCG is an invaluable part of monitoring the success of treating GTDs. Successful treatment sees the level drop from many thousands to almost zero. If the level rises again, the patient may have a recurrence. In addition to beta HCG, these tumours also put out loads of vasoactive peptides (VAPs). These are substances produced naturally during pregnancy to encourage the blood vessels supplying the uterus to grow in line with the growing uterus. You will remember we discussed earlier the uterine vessels enlarging from 2 to 3 mm in diameter to 10 mm; it is VAPs that make this happen. Other cancers also produce them as a way of getting themselves a new blood supply.

However, the trouble for us surgeons dealing with GTD is that the uterus takes on a huge blood supply, making serious bleeding during surgery much more likely. I remember well many years ago opening a woman to perform an urgent hysterectomy for a choriocarcinoma (she had completed her family, had a rapidly growing tumour, and was bleeding). When we looked in the abdomen, the anaesthetist, who was a locum, looked over and on seeing the size of the blood vessels, exclaimed, 'Are you really going to take that thing out?' He asked me to stop, whilst he inserted more intravenous lines. The ovarian and uterine vessels were all greater than a centimetre in diameter. It is partly looking after women in this situation that has stimulated such interest for me in how to control pelvic blood supply. These cases can be very scary.

Returning to PSTTs, they have a variable prognosis depending upon the time from the index pregnancy (the pregnancy that the disease arose from). PSTTs and ETTs secrete much lower beta HCG, and sometimes none at all, making it harder to monitor treatment progress. In contrast to other GTDs, PSTTs can arise from normal pregnancies as well as from a miscarriage or a mole. If a PSTT has come from a pregnancy in the last four years, then the prognosis, even in the presence of distant metastases, is excellent. However, if it's over five years, the picture is very different. A cure rate of over 80% drops to 20%. This makes for very difficult decision for women in this position who do not have a child, or who wish for more children. It is possible to genetically type these tumours and, if there is a child, to make comparison and see if the PSTT has arisen from that pregnancy. This is not possible with miscarriages, however, since there is no tissue to genetically type.

In the early 2000s, Michael Seckl and I had noted that amongst the women with PSTT, some had multiple sites of disease, but others had only one in the uterus. Following the success of the modified Strassman procedure in the woman with the giant adenomatoid tumour, we wondered if we could not do something similar in women with single-site PSTT in the uterus. The typical principle of all cancer surgery is to remove the tumour with 1 cm of normal tissue surrounding it. This makes local recurrence of the tumour very unlikely. The original plan was to open the patient's abdomen, isolate the blood supply to the uterus, to then use cutting diathermy — a standard piece of surgical equipment that looks like a needle, but with an electric current running through it to prevent bleeding. This does, of course, also cause thermal damage to the surrounding tissue to a depth of 2 to 3 mm — more on this soon! We cut into the uterus, found the tumour and then cut it out with a margin of normal uterine tissue around it. The tumour with surrounding normal tissue was then subjected to immediate analysis by histopathologist Dr Ian Lindsay; this technique is called frozen section (FS) analysis. Ian would determine whether there was tumour extending to the cut edge, or we had an appropriate margin of normal tissue. If the margin of normal tissue was not there, a hysterectomy would be performed. The patients were all fully informed of the possible risk of tumour spread by opening the uterus and not just removing the tumour intact in a hysterectomy case.

What we then found was that we sometimes were struggling to find the tumour. I come from the generation of gynaecologists where you were either a scanner or a surgeon, not both. Scanning was not at the front of my mind. However, my trainee at the time — my now-colleague and friend Mr Joseph Yazbek — had the great idea of aqua floating the pelvis — in other words, filling it with water — and then putting the ultrasound probe in a sterile bag and scanning the uterus to identify the tumour. A fantastic idea, and it worked.

Our next problem came as Ian rightly told us: our margins were too close on frozen section analysis, and we therefore removed the uterus only to discover that there was no tumour left when the final analysis of the specimen took place. This was because of the 2 to 3 mm of thermal damage from the cutting diathermy device, which made it look as though we were too close when we weren't. We therefore now use needle diathermy at the start when we are clear of the tumour, but swap back to an old-fashioned steel blade for the excision of the tumour, in the knowledge that what the pathologist gets is the real deal, with no thermal damage where it counts — i.e., abutting the tumour.

Appropriate approvals were sought, and over two to three years we performed five cases. In the first one no FS analysis was performed, but on later analysis of the margins, edges of the tumour were too close, and the patient underwent completion hysterectomy within two weeks. In the next two cases we had introduced FS, but the margins were positive upon FS analysis. An immediate hysterectomy was thus performed, but of these two hysterectomy samples, one had no disease, and the other did. This was when ultrasound was introduced. We then had another positive margin on FS, and immediate hysterectomy was performed, but there was no residual disease in the hysterectomy sample.

In other words, we had successfully removed the tumour in two out of four cases. But the diathermy artefact had misled us. In the final case, we used ultrasound identification of the tumour and a cold knife to excise it. The FS analysis of the tumour was negative, and this woman went on to have a baby.

Funnily enough, in the days of pagers, I was walking around the south end of the Isle of Bute on holiday when I was paged by Charing Cross switchboard. Unlike mobile phones, pagers worked everywhere except underground. Unusually, it was a patient calling me. My initial slight irritation turned to great joy as she told me who she was, and that lying beside her was her newborn baby. She was the first woman in the world to deliver a baby following fertility-sparing surgery for a PSTT. This was in the early 2000s, and again was further proof that you could block off the blood supply to the uterus and perform major surgery on it — even cutting it in half to just above the cervix — and if you performed a careful reconstruction, it would allow a successful pregnancy. From the transplant angle, of course, the uterus has no blood supply for hours. We finally published these results in 2012.

• Part III •
Progress and Surgery

5

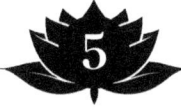

Endometrial Transplantation

A sherman's Syndrome is a form of infertility caused by adhesions, or scar tissue, within the uterine cavity. It affects up to 1.5% of the population and is the cause of 1 in 20 cases of infertility in women. It remains a poorly-understood condition, but is thought to arise following trauma to the basal layer of the endometrium, such as following a termination of pregnancy, or surgical evacuation of a miscarriage. The basal endometrium is the layer within the uterine cavity that is stimulated by hormones every month and then shed once the hormone levels reduce, causing a woman to have a period. Many women with Asherman's syndrome can undergo minor surgery to remove the scar tissue and normalise the cavity. However, women with severe cases may remain infertile.

The classic story of Asherman's syndrome is of a couple who start trying for a baby. Very happily, the woman falls pregnant, but sadly, at 8 weeks, she goes for a scan and it transpires she has lost the baby. She is admitted for a minor but distressing surgical procedure to empty the uterus. All goes well and she is discharged home the same day. The weeks go by, and she has only a very light period or no period at all. She is, however, still having a hormonal cycle, as women with MRKH do. She is re-referred to the gynaecology department and another scan is performed, which finds that the endometrium (the lining of the womb) is too thin. A procedure follows to look inside the womb and instead of a nice healthy cavity, there are adhesions (synechiae), whereby it's all stuck together. There are various treatments possible, but they often fail. The result is infertility not treatable by any known method apart from transplanting a new uterus into the woman, even though the remainder of her uterus is normal. There are also women who do fall pregnant again, but go on to have multiple miscarriages – again, extremely distressing. The final subgroup in this scenario consists of those who do fall pregnant, but this time around, the afterbirth, instead of sticking normally to the wall on the inside of the uterus, grows through it. This is extremely dangerous. To illustrate this, here follows a true story.

A great friend and colleague of Richard's, Professor Mark Johnston, asked him to come to the Labour Ward at Chelsea and Westminster Hospital in London to help with a case. There was a woman at 38 weeks pregnant, and she had her placenta growing though her uterus into her bladder. She required a Caesarean section and possibly a hysterectomy. A hysterectomy in this circumstance could not use a bikini incision but instead required an up-and-down, and thus general anaesthesia. There followed the first problem: the patient had a short thick neck, and it took three consultant anaesthetists to intubate her, with Dr Viv Thomas saving the day. She was then opened through this up-and-down midline incision, and her baby was safely delivered through the top of her uterus, well away from the placenta. Looking to the bottom of the uterus, one could see the placenta lurking there surrounded by huge vessels. The dome (top) of the bladder was also involved. The uterus was sutured and closed.

A debate then ensued about whether to leave the placenta to die away on its own with a substantial risk of haemorrhage in the next 24 hours, or remove the uterus there and then. That quandary was solved when the anaesthetist, the late Dr Peter Barnes, informed the team that if she bled later, she would die, because they would not be able to get a tube into her lungs again in the near future. The decision was made, and in about two hours, the entire blood supply to the uterus had been isolated, except where the bladder was involved. This is seriously scary surgery, bad for the coronary arteries! The anaesthetists, who had a pump so they could rapidly get blood into the woman, were informed that that this was the point where the uterus had to come out, and to expect brisk bleeding. The uterus came out in under one minute. She lost six pints of blood in that short time – but it was all replaced within a few minutes.

So how could we prevent this sort of nightmare? This is where the new biomaterials we are developing, along with work on endometrial transplantation, come in – potentially life-changing and life-giving. The panoply of issues relating to Asherman's can seem enormous. The question is: Could a procedure be developed which is less invasive and risky than uterine transplantation for this group? This chapter and the next will address our work in this area.

The original idea to transplant the endometrium came from Professor Yau Thum, our infertility advisor. He had done his PhD a few years prior on natural killer cells, their function in the endometrium, and their role in infertility. Moreover, in our experience in gynaecological surgery, the endometrium can be repaired by suturing it back onto the muscle layer of the uterus. This is evident following removal of fibroids, or after the previously described modified Strassman procedure, when entering the cavity is unavoidable. One uterine transplantation case had been undertaken for severe Asherman's syndrome; we proposed endometrial transplantation as a less-invasive option. This work formed part of Ben's PhD, and has some symbiosis with Maxine's work in tissue engineering, which, as you will see in Chapter 6, has concentrated on the endometrium rather than the rest of the uterus. Further work was undertaken by Saaliha (Sal) Vali, one of our current Research Fellows, in this area which is also presented later.

Ben and Richard contacted Professor Noakes at the Royal Veterinary College and looked at a few cadaveric animal uteri to decide how to run our project. We decided that rabbits were the best model and reached out to Professor Paco Jimenez in Valencia. The main rationale for using rabbits was that female rabbits have a duplex uterus, with two separate uterine horns and two cervices. This makes them an ideal candidate for reproductive studies, as they have an in-built control horn that can be used to compare against the operated horn. In addition, our research team also has extensive experience in operating on the rabbit pelvis, due to previous uterine transplant studies undertaken in the past.

So, in January 2018, Ben, Isabel (who had been brought on board in 2014) and Richard took off for Spain to work with our old friend and collaborator Paco and his colleagues. The British press make much play of the UK's superiority in our scientific establishments; a trip to Valencia is a good way to dispel that myth. Their facilities and standards are exemplary. We had performed a preliminary project that had proved it was technically possible to remove the endometrium in a rabbit. We had also gained important knowledge of the blood supply to the uterus, and established a way to temporarily reduce blood supply to it using metal clips to reduce blood loss whilst we operated. We worked out that there was a significant variation in the size of the uterus depending on where the rabbit was on its cycle; the size was optimal for the purposes of removing and reimplanting the endometrium in the five days following ovulation.

We arrived in Valencia late on Sunday night. After a cramped EasyJet flight, we decided to get an early night in anticipation for an early start the following day. Paco collected us first thing in the morning, and we were greeted at the facility at the Valencia Polytechnic University by the rest of his team. The rabbits had had ovulation induced five days prior and had been acclimatised to their new surroundings.

We performed three endometrial transplants on the first day. The learning curve was steep, and the fluidity and economy of our movement improved with each operation, which resulted in faster procedures. That evening we were treated to a beautiful meal of traditional Valencian paella. It was hands-down the best paella we'd ever tasted, although this version contained rabbit, which was ironic and morbid considering we'd spent all day trying to keep our rabbits alive!

Over the three days we performed 10 operations. We performed eight endometrial auto-transplants, which incorporated removing the lining of the womb, placing it into cold perfusion solution, and then reimplanting it, before closing the uterus. We also performed two cases where we removed only the lining of the womb, and did not reimplant it with the intention that this would control against the endometrium regeneration. Unfortunately, despite our best efforts, two rabbits from the transplant group died during the operations, one due to anaesthetic-related issues, and the other due to excessive bleeding, which contributed to our difficulty in adjusting anaesthetic doses. Three rabbits were euthanised 48, 72, and 96 hours post-op to assess the how the lining of the uterus was reimplanting into the muscle layer beneath. These were assessed under high magnification, which demonstrated that the tissue looked viable and operation thus possible. We monitored the remaining five rabbits closely after the operations and looked after them as they recovered. Unfortunately, two rabbits, one from the transplant group and one from the control group, died four weeks and eight weeks after, respectively, for reasons we could not determine. Three rabbits subsequently underwent embryo transfer, and all three subsequently became pregnant. In the uterus that was not operated on, 57% of embryos implanted; in the operated uteri of the two rabbits that had endometrium transplanted, the implantation rate was 28.5%. In the operated uterus of the control rabbit where the endometrium was removed, no pregnancies were achieved. Despite successful implantations in the transplanted uteri, pregnancies did not develop, and sadly no live births were achieved.

A further embryo transfer cycle was carried out, with similar results. Following euthanasia of the remaining rabbits, the endometrium looked viable both to the naked eye and when assessed under high magnification. Whilst the operation was successful, unfortunately the lack of live births brought us to the conclusion that whilst the blood supply was sufficient to allow the endometrium to reimplant, it was not enough to support a growing pregnancy. As we have seen time and time again, such as in the first human uterus transplant, novel surgical techniques are rarely a success the first time. However, the enormous lessons learned during this study brought us hope that with further refinement, this could be an option for women with Asherman's syndrome in the future.

To this end, we (Sal, Maxine, Ben, Isabel and Richard) returned to Valencia in March 2022 to see if we could improve our results in the transplanted endometrium by utilising protein rich plasma (PRP) or microfragmented adipose fat (MFAT). The former technique involves centrifuging blood and injecting the PRP into the endometrium. MFAT is collected by a liposuction technique, the likes of which is used by plastic surgeons removing fat from the abdominal wall. This work therefore tested two hypotheses:

1. PRP will recruit endogenous stem cells, which will differentiate and form new vessels, improving blood flow and inducing healing of the re-transplanted endometrium, leading to improved IVF outcomes.
2. MFAT will recruit endogenous stem cells, which will differentiate and form new vessels improving blood flow and inducing healing of the re-transplanted endometrium, leading to improved IVF outcomes.

The results proved interesting. As a quick refresher, a rabbit's uterus has two long arms, or horns, where the pups grow and the arms join centrally over the single cervix and vagina.

As with our 2018 trial, in each subject one side of the uterus was transplanted and the other was left untouched as a control. A month after the transplantation of the endometrium, embryo transfer was undertaken. Laparoscopy was undertaken two weeks later to assess for implantation. The implantation rate was 63%, compared to 4% in the control arm. In the 2018 project without PRP or MFAT, the implanta-tion rate was 28.5%.

Writing now in 2024, it is clear this work needs to be revisited. As a team we have rightly been concentrating on transplanting uteruses in a human setting. However, the relative success of these two projects, coupled with Maxine Chan's work described in the next chapter, shows that we should combine the strengths of both works and resume work in this area.

Chapter

6

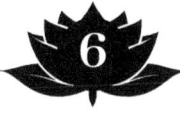

Tissue Engineering

About 20 years ago, I went literally round the corner from my office at the Chelsea and Westminster Hospital to see the Professor of Tissue Engineering at that time, Julia Pollak (now sadly deceased). I told her about my research and then said to her, 'I am embarrassed to even suggest it, but could you grow a uterus?' She replied, 'You go show you can transplant one, and come back and talk to me.'

About 16 years later I was able to come back having fulfilled Julia's challenge, but sadly she was gone, and I reached out to her successor, Professor Dame Molly Stevens DBE FRS. We met, and to my great joy she accepted one of our fellows into her group, the first gynaecologist to join that illustrious band of scientists. This was great luck, compounded for us by finding Dr Maxine Chan, a very smart Research Fellow, who happily has blossomed in Molly's group. There are few gynaecologists who could or would have swum in this high-science environment; it's just as well that I wasn't applying for the job! These projects are supported by another charity, Wellbeing of Women.

Before diving into the detail of the valuable work being undertaken by Maxine and Molly, a bit of further context is needed to explain the issue their research addresses. Earlier (page 59) with the evacuation of the uterus, you might be forgiven for thinking that perhaps the method of emptying the uterus was performed incompetently. Very occasionally that might be the case, but more likely it's down to the way a particular woman's body heals; unfortunately, that person has an endometrium, that forms excessive scar tissue.

This is analogous to three patients having a similar operation. One forms minimal scar tissue at the skin – a good scar, in other words; us surgeons are very good at taking credit for those wounds. The second person will form moderate scar tissue, and unfortunately another the third will form dense scar tissue, known a keloid, on the skin. Surgeons then tend to blame the patient, not the technique. Dense scar tissue post-surgery on the skin often reflects what is going inside, and this can have devastating consequences. The same type of thing can happen in the benign, non-cancerous condition of endometriosis. Most women with this condition, where the lining of the womb lies outside the womb, will have fairly minimal symptoms, but there is also a sub-group whose lives have been wrecked by this condition.

Again, you might be forgiven for thinking that the creation of scar tissue is down to surgical technique. There is no doubting that meticulous surgery is better than rough surgery, but most of the time it is probably the patient's bodily response that at least partly determines the outcome.

In the last couple of decades, it has now been recognised that in most diseases such as cancer and organ failure that it is damage to the tissue microenvironment that makes repair an unfavourable prospect. Bioengineering applies natural principles of biology to addressing a medical issue, such as correcting inappropriate biological responses in individuals. Our research instead takes the unique approach of harnessing and utilising the natural properties of tissue matrix proteins to tackle scarring inside the uterus and stimulate healthy endometrial repair. This is an example of biomimicry – taking inspiration from nature to create solutions to human challenges.

Asherman's syndrome has been thoroughly described in the previous chapter. The RCOG report that adhesions form in up to 18.5% of women who have had surgical management of miscarriage, with

42% of those being moderate to severe adhesions. Adhesions are an important cause of absolute uterine factor infertility and the prevalence of adhesions amongst women with infertility has been reported to be as high has 22%. They can also be a cause of recurrent miscarriage and abnormal placental attachment. For women with infertility secondary to adhesions, there are limited treatment options. Current preventative treatments for adhesions have low or variable efficacy, and there are no therapies that specifically target fibrosis. The aim of our research was to develop novel bioengineering strategies by way of biogels (also called hydrogels) to prevent intrauterine scarring and promote the regeneration of a healthy endometrium – and in so doing, provide better treatment options for women with uterine factor infertility.

It is important to remember that what we are about is the relief of suffering. This takes place in the relief of pain, the treatment of infertility, and thus the begetting of children – all such important components of human flourishing. When you see the consequences for these women, who are currently in a terrible place with long-term pain and suffering, coupled with the inability to have children, and then look to what we are trying to achieve, this research really has the capacity to benefit millions of women worldwide. Our recent calculations suggest that if this treatment is successful, and if this biogel came to be utilised in all women having an evacuation of uterus post-miscarriage, it would prevent 70,000 cases of Asherman's syndrome per year in the UK alone.

Ironically, when Maxine started, the goal had been to try to construct a whole uterus – but the decision was rapidly made that concentrating on the endometrium would lead to faster results benefiting a larger number of women. Molly was of the view that fully constructing a uterus would be a 15-to-20-year project.

The remainder of this chapter consists of selected extracts from Maxine's thesis conclusions, as I don't think I can summarise any better. Maxine has produced a superb thesis of high science running to 270 pages. Her thesis is now published, and much of it in print, for those that are interested in the details. I have modified her conclusions to those which seemed most salient to me as a practising physician, and thus I hope, our readers.

> 'Intrauterine scarring is an important cause of infertility and other pregnancy complications, for which current treatments are not highly effective. In recent years there has been a growing trend in studying regenerative medicine approaches to treating a damaged or scarred endometrium. The aim of this thesis was to explore a biomaterials approach to endometrial repair, by developing and characterising an endometrial extra cellular matrix (ECM) hydrogel which was hypothesised to have favourable material and biological properties to mitigate intrauterine fibrosis and support endometrial regeneration.
>
> In this project, a novel method for decellularising porcine endometrial tissue was described and it was demonstrated that key ECM proteins and proteoglycans were preserved in the decellularised endometrial ECM. Matrix-bound nanovesicles, with exosome-like properties, were found within the decellularised endometrial ECM. This has not been reported before in other studies on de-cellularised reproductive tissues. An endometrial ECM hydrogel was demonstrated to be injectable and sprayable and, like all ECM hydrogels, gelation was initiated within minutes under physiological conditions. These properties make the ECM hydrogel versatile for in vivo applications, in other words potentially translatable into clinical practice.
>
> Endometrial ECM hydrogel was shown to have good cellular compatibility and led to increased vessel growth (angiogenesis *in vitro*) also suggesting a potential beneficial modulatory effect on the immune system thus potentially assisting when it comes to wound healing.'

Future Work

> 'To further develop the understanding of the properties and bioactivity of endometrial ECM (extracellular matrix) hydrogel, future studies could involve investigating the modulatory properties of the immune system in endometrial Matrix Bound Nanovesicles

(MBVs), and to characterise the effect of endometrial ECM on stem cells. It would also be important to understand the similarities and differences between endometrial ECM and other ECM types in the context of endometrial regeneration to appreciate whether there is a tissue-specific advantage. The *in vivo* work presented in this thesis focused on primary prevention of intrauterine fibrosis. Further experimental work would include determining the effect of endometrial ECM hydrogel in the treatment of existing intrauterine scarring. If future studies could demonstrate the efficacy of endometrial ECM gel, alone, for endometrial regeneration and fertility restoration, this would be a significant improvement on the one existing animal study on endometrial ECM gel which found beneficial effects only when ECM was combined with growth factor delivery. This is an especially important consideration for moving this into the clinical setting. Whilst ECM hydrogels have been used to deliver drugs, growth factors and cells, the addition of these extra components increases the cost and complexity of manufacture and may limit the stability or shelf-life of the treatment.

The eventual goal of this research is to progress closer towards the clinical setting, with a gel that can be easily applied in a surgical setting for primary or secondary prevention of intrauterine adhesions and promotion of functional endometrial regeneration. Endometrial function is ultimately defined by fertility and maintenance of pregnancy. Therefore, future work would benefit from the investigation of pregnancy outcome when endometrial ECM hydrogel has been used to prevent or treat a damaged endometrium.'

Contextualisation of This Research

'The use of hydrogels to prevent or treat adhesions in the uterus is a growing field. Hyaluronic acid (HA) gels are already used clinically for prevention of these adhesions, as well as pelvic adhesions after abdominal surgery. They have been demonstrated to reduce adhesion formation, but their efficacy for improving fertility and pregnancy rates is still unproven clinically. HA hydrogel could be used as a control in future studies. However, to select an appropriate control, a clinically approved, commercially manufactured HA would be necessary. This thesis was inspired by the observation of the uncertain impact of existing clinical therapies on pregnancy outcomes and by appraising studies on decellularised uterine tissue, which showed favourable effects on uterine regeneration and fertility restoration in animal studies. These studies suggested that there were tissue-specific advantages to using uterine ECM for endometrial repair. The recent studies by another group on the development of an endometrial ECM hydrogel for intended treatment of Asherman's syndrome and endometrial atrophy further validated the concept of designing a novel, tissue-specific approach to endometrial regeneration that may ultimately prove to be superior to existing therapies for restoring fertility. The results presented in this work suggested many favourable properties of ECM hydrogels for constructive tissue healing. However, this type of biomaterial has some important considerations to be borne in mind before entering the clinical arena. Research and development focus must be given to minimising batch-to-batch variability in ECM biomaterials. Decellularised ECM is a highly complex material biochemically and there needs to be greater emphasis on developing ways to ensure or evaluate for uniformity, compared to hydrogels that are made from one compound or that are chemically synthesised. The mechanical properties of an ECM hydrogel could be made more consistent by incorporating cross-linkers or mixing with another type of hydrogel. Another consideration for clinical translation is that there still remains a lack of standardisation as to what degree of cell and DNA removal is safe and what biochemical components are essential to be preserved in ECM biomaterials in order for them to be effective. Reducing this ambiguity would improve the quality and efficacy of ECM hydrogels, ultimately resulting in more robust clinical responses.'

Implications for Other Areas of Research

'Whilst the emphasis of this thesis was on intrauterine scarring, the findings generated by this work have implications for other clinical diseases that affect female reproductive health. Adhesions in the pelvis, outside of the uterus, form commonly after abdominal and pelvic surgery or as a result of endometriosis. Pelvic adhesions can cause pain, infertility and surgical complications, but a recent review found no evidence of the effectiveness of current anti-adhesion therapies for improving pelvic pain or pregnancy outcomes. It would be interesting to investigate whether endometrial ECM hydrogel could also mitigate fibrosis in pelvic adhesions. Endometrial atrophy can occur in conjunction with Asherman's syndrome or as a result of uterine surgery, radiotherapy, infection or of unknown cause. A thin endometrium results in lower pregnancy and live birth rates during assisted reproduction and there are limited effective treatments. Endometrial ECM hydrogel was demonstrated to improve endometrial cell growth and increase blood vessel growth in this work. Therefore, there is the potential for endometrial ECM hydrogel to be investigated as a treatment for regenerating atrophic endometrium. Enhancing cell proliferation and blood vessel growth are desirable traits for tissue regeneration and whilst these same biological processes are also implicated in cancer development and progression, this author has identified no reports regarding cancer risk associated with ECM biomaterials. It would be very interesting to explore, in future, the role of ECM hydrogels as an adjunctive treatment in gynaecological cancers, either in the prevention of scarring and cancer progression following surgical removal of disease or potentially as a combination therapy with progesterone in the management of early-stage endometrial cancer when fertility-sparing treatment is desired.

The work presented in this thesis involved the development, characterisation and application of an endometrial ECM hydrogel produced in a novel way. Overall, the results indicated the beneficial effect of endometrial ECM hydrogel for preventing fibrosis and supporting biological processes that are important for tissue regeneration. The in vivo work was promising for the ability of endometrial ECM hydrogel to limit endometrial damage after injury. These findings pave the way for more research to understand the impact of endometrial ECM hydrogel for treating established intrauterine scarring and for fertility restoration.'

Concluding Remark from Richard

I, for one, believe this research to be the project of all projects associated with Womb Transplant UK which will influence the most people before all is said and done. It was for this reason that the Garfield Weston Foundation agreed to fund work with Molly, Srdjan, Maxine and myself in this area.

Chapter

7

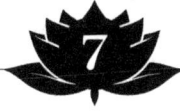

Uterine Transplantation Breakthroughs

In October 2014, I had an unforgettable day. I had been in Bristol lecturing and, for the first time ever, was not greeted with hostility from at least some of the audience for our projected project. I phoned Srdjan from the train as I returned to London to tell him this good news. It was only then that I was phoned with the astounding news that the Swedish group had success with the delivery of a live baby at 32 weeks gestation by Caesarean section from a woman who had a transplanted uterus. What they (and by they, I mean the woman who had the transplant, the woman who donated the uterus, and the surgical team lead by Mats Brännström) had achieved was incredible, and really brave on all their parts.

The various groups — Swedish, American and ourselves — had all been circling round the possibility for years, but until it was done, one could never know if it would actually work. People used to ask if we wanted to be first, but we didn't deserve that; we had fallen behind Mats and his group by about two or three years and were not ready to apply for Ethics until 2015. When I was reading Srdjan's PhD prior to its submission (he passed!), I realised that Mats and his group in 2013 had published 70 peer-reviewed publications, a total that we only reached in two years later. At this point we applied for, and were granted, permission by a National Ethics committee to perform 10 DBD uterine transplants. So why did so many years go by until we moved over the line? Here lies a tale to which my fellow between 2015 and 2019, Ben Jones, contributed much. I will confess that at the time, I had a great naivety about the process which would ensue.

Deceased Donor Donation, Autumn 2022

Our goal all along had been to set up a sustainable national uterine transplant programme. In 2015, our team believed that to be sustainable, we needed to go down the cadaveric, or deceased donor, route. Our rationale for this was based on our experience from the original transplant cases, wherein retrieval from living donors took 10 to 13 hours. The length of time a patient is on the operating table partly determines the risk of deep venous thrombosis (DVT). DVT is clot formation in the leg that can break off and travel to the lungs, a condition known as pulmonary embolism (PE) or venous thromboembolism (VTE), which can result in death of part of the lung and, with particularly large clots, the death of the patient. It is known that operations lasting over 6 hours carry increased risk of VTE with each succeeding hour. Clearly, with deceased donation, there are no such worries. As such, we put all our effort into constructing a deceased-donor trial, leading, we hope, to a NHS sustainable uterine transplant programme.

To be able to plug into the national DBD programme rightly requires much regulatory process. It is vitally important that we gynaecologists do nothing to harm the national multi-organ retrieval programme, which is so important for those waiting for new hearts, lungs, kidneys, livers, pancreas and small bowel — all organs vital to survival. Additionally, it is essential to have the approval of specialist nurses in organ donation (SNOD), as they are the people who talk to donor families, and intensivists (anaesthetists running intensive care units where the donors will be cared for). We also needed approval to retrieve the uterus from the Human Tissue Authority (HTA), which entailed an enormity of documents and protocols.

Between 2016 and late 2018, we also met with the regulatory committees within NHS Blood and Transplantation (NHSBT); the National Retrieval Group (NRG), a multidisciplinary group of healthcare professionals involved in the multi-organ retrieval process; the Research Innovation and Novel Technologies group (RINTAG), a committee that approves novel or research techniques; and the National Organ Donation Committee (NODC), another multi-disciplinary group that regulates organ donation. We were also quite correctly required to have the Royal College of Obstetricians and Gynaecologists (RCOG) on board. This involved presenting to their Scientific Advisory Committee on a number of occasions over the years, as well as meeting the successive RCOG Presidents, nearly all of whom have been supportive over the years. It was only following the approval of all these sub-committees that the NHSBT Senior Management Committee finally gave us their own approval on 15th January 2019. Because it had taken so long to achieve NHSBT approval, we were required to re-submit for Ethics approval. It's also important to point out that the failure of any of these submissions would result in overall failure, so there have been some very stressful moments as we wound through this process.

We had our retrieval team set up and had done cadaveric retrievals. Myself, Isabel, Ben, Sal, supported by colleagues Cesar Diaz-Garcia, Srdjan Saso, Ahmad Sayasneh, Sadaf Ghaem-Maghami, and Jay Chatterjee, all gynaecological cancer surgeons, are all officially ticketed as organ retrievers. Isabel, Venkatesha, Ben and myself are the implanters. The team structure has evolved as our programme has developed. We realised that before enlarging the team, we needed to have a core team who acquired the appropriate skills. Isabel and Sadaf saw this development far more clearly than I did. The current core team structure has me leading the retrieval, assisted by Isabel and Ben and either Fellow, Sal or Ari. The back table work to make the uterus transplantable is led by Isabel, assisted by her transplant colleagues — Venkatesha, Ann (the transplant specialist trainee) Ben and myself. Venkatesha was originally assisted by Saso or myself when opening the recipient but is now assisted by transplant colleagues. Then Ben and I remove the vestiges of the uterus and Fallopian tubes in the MRKH cases, or the uterus if it is non-functional. Thereafter, Isabel returns to the table, and performs the vessel anastomosis with Venkatesha. This is the most complicated part of the procedure. Ben and I then do the stitching-in of the uterus, with its cuff of vagina, to the vagina of the recipient, and then create the ligamentous support.

In 2016, we registered our project long-term with NHS England with the goal of having an NHS-funded centre in future. This four-year process, which was designed to run in tandem with our four-year research programme, has of course extended out to eight years so far, with the expectation of completion in late 2026. Much work is ongoing in this area, and we are hopeful that we will obtain this funding for our DBD programme.

Meanwhile, all our funding is charitable via Womb Transplant UK. This, as we mentioned earlier, is a charity designed to fund, in full, the first ten deceased-donor research transplants without cost to the NHS. It has also pledged to fund five living-donor transplants. For 25 years, we were funded on a shoestring with no input from the NHS or from large funding bodies. We were supported only by fundraising events, two small charities, a number of individuals, and small grants from the industry. This changed dramatically for us with our two new patrons Nick and Nadine in 2022. Neil Huband has guided us all through the media minefield with great skill and no fees charged. All of our doctors, nurses, and veterinarians have never received a penny in recompense for their efforts, which for many have been enormous. Only the sequential Fellows have received a salary; as they are Medical Officers in HCA hospitals, their work with transplant has also been pro bono. We have also been fortunate enough to have been the Lister Hospital's designated charity since 2014.[7]

---

[7] Lister Fertility, under the Directorship of Sam Abdalla for many years and now James Nicopoullos, and in the skilful hands of Yau Thum and Ben, are performing the IVF which includes preimplantation genetic testing to minimise the risks of any of the pregnancies going wrong.

Live Donation Breakthrough

The sea change for us came at a conference in Gothenburg in 2017. At the conference dinner, Isabel, Ben and I were lucky to sit with Liza Johannesson and Giuliano Testa. Liza is a Professor of Gynaecology and worked on the original Swedish programme with Mats. Giuliano is a transplant surgeon, and they work together with their team at Baylor University Medical Center in Dallas, Texas, in the US, running what is currently the world's largest living-donor uterine transplant programme. Stina Jarvholm, a Swedish psychologist who rendered much help to our programme back in 2015, was also dining with us. Liza described a new approach to live-donor retrieval which, I must confess, I did not grasp that evening. However, the following day Liza expanded on her approach when she gave her talk. This was a genuine 'wow' moment. Liza's retrieval did away with the original technique of dissecting out the internal iliac arteries and veins – a long and tricky process – and instead utilised the internal iliac arteries and provided drainage via the ovarian veins. In an irony of ironies, our radical trachelectomy 20 years earlier had led us to the possibility of uterine transplant, and now here we were, round in one huge circle, to an effectively modified radical abdominal trachelectomy retrieval. This allowed us to look seriously at a living-donor programme. Remember that at trachelectomy, the uterus is supplied by the ovarian arteries and drained via the ovarian veins. During the trachelectomy procedure, we do, however, dissect the uterine vessels and the internal iliac arteries.

My realisation during Liza's talk – that I had failed to see the obvious – was so startling to me that I had to run down the steps of the lecture theatre to catch Liza and confirm that I had understood correctly. We now could see a way toward retrievals in living donors below the six-hour threshold. This propelled us down a concurrent live-donor programme as well as our deceased-donor programme, which at the time was already well advanced in terms of approvals. Over the ensuing years Liza and Giuliano's new methodology has been proven to work, and they graciously invited us out to Dallas and agreed to be our collaborators for the first living-donor transplants. We visited them in the spring of 2019.

The following illustrations show the original method of retrieval incorporating the internal iliac arteries and veins.

In Figure 7.1, we see on the left the original retrieval in the Swedish living donor programme. This is the same retrieval we have used in our deceased donor programme. On the right, the figure shows the graft encompassing the uterus, a cuff of vagina, Fallopian tubes, uterine arteries and veins leading to the internal iliac arteries and vein.

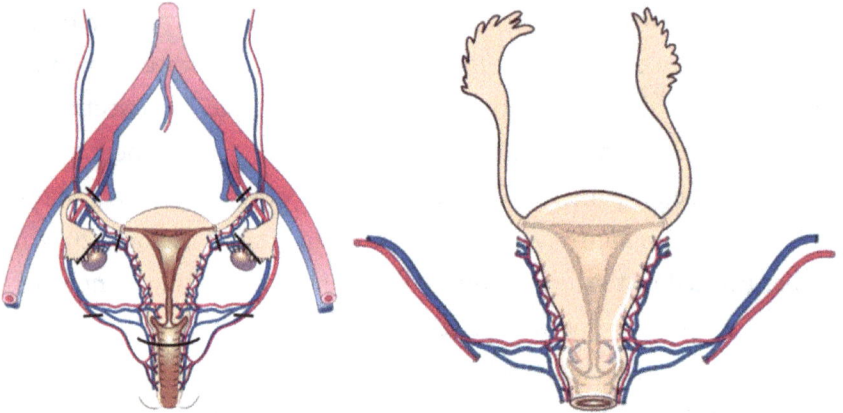

Figure 7.1. Complex uteric/venous dissection.

Next, the graft is inserted, with the internal iliac arteries and veins now stitched onto the external iliac vessels in the recipient (Figure 7.2). The vagina has also been sutured.

Figure 7.3 shows the graft obtained by the new Dallas retrieval method, with uterus, vaginal cuff, Fallopian tubes, uterine arteries, internal iliac arteries, and ovarian veins. The vital difference, which ultimately led us to adopt living donation, is that the venous drainage (veins returning deoxygenated blood to the heart) is via the ovarian vessels, thus greatly reducing operative retrieval times in living donors.

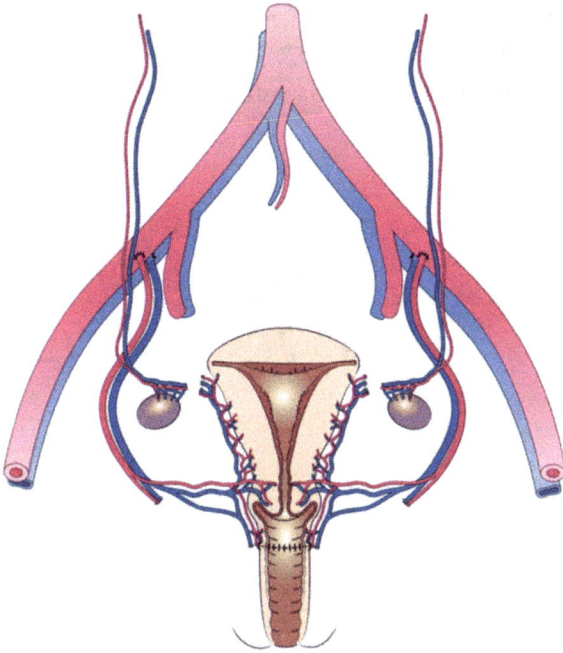

Figure 7.2. Deceased donor graft inserted into recipient.

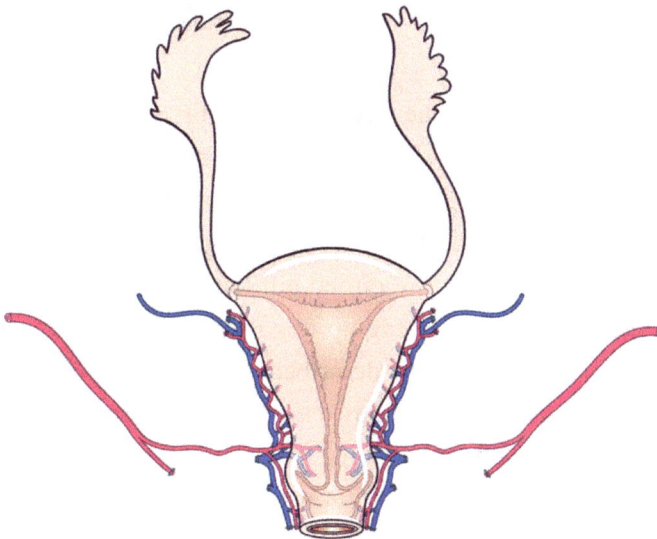

Figure 7.3. Dallas retrieval method.

The graft is implanted (Figure 7.4), with the internal iliac vessels sutured to the external iliac artery, the ovarian veins sutured to the external iliac veins, and the vagina sutured.

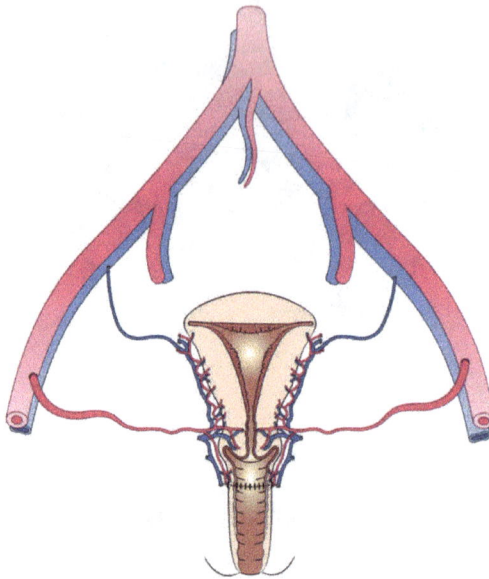

Figure 7.4. Transplanted uterus in the recipient, utilising the iliac and ovarian vessels.

We managed to add the new living donor programme relatively rapidly, assisted by the fact that this is now an established procedure in the US, and that our teams have extensive experience of performing abdominal radical trachelectomy in the management of cervical cancer. It was from this point that 'we girded our loins' and really got down to the recruitment process, gearing up to go as we ploughed through the permissions process previously described.

One new result of our announcement that we proposed to undertake a living-donor transplant programme was that many hundreds of women emailed us looking to donate their uteruses. At that time, we were primarily focussed on related donor–recipient pairings for the living-donor programme, that is, sister to sister, or mother to daughter.

In response to the huge surge in potential altruistic donors, Ben undertook a fascinating study on 150 women in order to better understand the huge group of women looking to donate altruistically to an unknown recipient. He concluded that more than 97% of respondents simply wished to donate their uterus to help other women carry their own baby, and 97% no longer needed their womb. After being informed in more detail of the risks inherent in the process, 95% were still keen to donate. However, once the donor selection criteria were applied, only 27% were suitable to proceed. This group may become significant as we explore possibilities to open an altruistic-donor programme in the future.

Eligibility Criteria for Deceased and Living Donor Transplant Recipients

The criteria annotated describe those drawn up for our deceased donor trial. It is well accepted that these criteria will widen in future. These criteria related to the recipient are as follows:

- Absolute uterine factor infertility
- 24 to 42 years of age
- No intercurrent medical condition
- Body Mass Index (BMI) not high
- Accepting of having one or two children and of having a hysterectomy on completion of their family
- Have embryos already created from one's own eggs by IVF and in cold storage
- No pelvic kidney
- A reasonable length of vagina that has not been constructed from non-vaginal tissue (e.g., bowel).

The criteria for deceased donors are:

- 18 to 50 years of age
- Normal uterine morphology on ultrasound
- Having previously delivered babies

- Having had not more than two Caesarean sections
- Testing negative for HPV
- Testing negative for sexually transmitted infections

The criteria for living donors are:

- Between 30 and 55 years of age, with the upper limit related to menopausal status
- Normal uterine morphology
- Having previously had babies
- Fully counselled and independently assessed, with no evidence of coercion
- Fit to have major surgery
- No intercurrent medical conditions
- Testing negative for HPV
- Testing negative for sexually transmitted infections

Returning to our team's story, our permissions were in place and our protocols complete, and we were gearing up to commence our deceased-donor programme in January 2020. We had also planned our first living-donor transplant for March 2020. However, as outlined in the introduction, the stars were not aligned in our favour. In January and February, we were called six times for potential deceased donations, but none of the candidates were suitable. Then in early March, the first reports of COVID-19 began to appear. A friend who is a senior General Practitioner had been informed that it was expected that 500,000 people in the UK would die; landfill sites had been purchased. An anaesthetic colleague had a friend in Lombardy, Italy, who related the incredibly fast spread of infection and high death rate, particularly amongst the middle-aged and elderly.

Our practise run on 12th March was in fact a radical hysterectomy for a rare type of tumour, the operation being similar to a uterine transplant retrieval. There had been some joking at the operating table about dry coughs; little did we realise where things were going. After completing the procedure in the late afternoon, all consultants in the

Hammersmith theatre suite were called into the coffee room. There were probably about 40 of us – surgeons, anaesthetists and nurses.

Three senior managers and consultants then announced that theatres were going to be closed to turn the whole floor into one giant Intensive Care Unit (ITU). Hammersmith normally has two ITUs on either side of the theatre complex. It was then explained that we would all be re-detailed to work within this. Then the real sting in the tail came: if you contracted COVID-19 and were over the age of 60, you would be denied an ITU bed if you needed one – i.e., left to die! I had had my 60th birthday two months earlier – very bad timing indeed. Worse, within a day or so, of the team that had been in theatre on the 12th March, the two staff nurses, the healthcare assistant (HCA), registrar, consultant anaesthetist and myself all had high fevers, and retired to our beds. The staff nurses were young and recovered quickly. The HCA, anaesthetist and I sadly followed a different trajectory.

In all of this, there was one shaft of humour relating to the charity. Ben required a signature on a cheque, and so duly came to my abode, a permanently moored houseboat. I was very unwell, with raging temperatures, but this was at the beginning of the pandemic when there was no testing. The big plan was that he would place the cheque on the gangway, reverse off the gangway to a safe distance, and I, with gelled hands, would open the door, take the cheque, sign it, place it back on the gangway, and close the door: job done. When I ultimately opened the door, literally lathered in sweat with my nightclothes stuck to me, Ben was still on the gangway. He leapt backwards like a jack-in-the-box, with the words, 'You've really got it!' Too true.

The following blog post was written three days after I was discharged from hospital, on 30th March, 2020. It was of its moment, and the statistics are now much-modified in line with increasing under-standing of the disease. We have included it because it does form part of the story of Womb Transplant UK.

'On the 22 March 2020 I received an email from David Maloney, publisher at Darton, Longman and Todd, requesting whether his authors, of which I count it a great honour to be one, could perhaps contribute a piece for the internet during these dark and difficult times. Sadly, at the time I was in the COVID-19 isolation ward at the Chelsea and Westminster Hospital in London, on multiple antibiotics, oxygen and IV fluids. The question was whether I was lying there or dying there? Thankfully, I have been lucky and I was not dying – hence being able to write this piece.

I write as both a cancer surgeon and scientist. I, like so many of us, had many plans for this spring – long distance walks peppered with staying in good hotels – all of which were of course were swept away. Just over two weeks ago there was much joking in the operating theatre that we all had dry coughs; then a shortness of breath started the following day, and another 24 hours later high temperatures. I stayed at home alone and isolated for six days. Instead of my much-prayed-for deliverance things went from bad to worse, and I became confused. A friend picked up on this over the phone and pushed me to go to the hospital, a very fine piece of advice; my oxygen levels, as he had correctly surmised, were inadequate.

That morning as I left my home I wondered if I would ever see it again, but far worse was the isolation of knowing I might never see any of my four children ever again. This is the truly awful aspect of this virus; you die alone, with no visitors allowed, no farewells, no touch of the hand, no hugs, just the desert of an isolation ward. There are no faces, only masks.

Through all of this smell and taste are removed, and even worse the rare condition of dysgeusia. I had never heard of it before, but it is that condition in which things that should taste good are truly awful, enough to make you spit out your food and brush your teeth to get rid of the awful flavour. So, you eat nothing for days on end. This all goes along with wild hallucinations which go on all night, usually involving some fixed ideation around drowning in ones' own sweat and secretions. These would feel like dreams, then one would wake up lathered in sweat and breathless, only to plunge again and again into the same nightmare.

As a doctor, of course I am also obsessed with statistics. Now the COVID-19 story we all know is three percent mortality, not terrible, but not great, and really bad if you are in the three percent. However, this belies some truths; if you are thirty five years old and healthy, your chance of mortality is less than 0.1 percent. If you're sixty, you hit one percent. But at the point you go to hospital with pneumonia and a bit of adult respiratory distress syndrome (ARDS), it goes up to between five and ten percent; if you are on a ventilator it increases to over fifty percent. To put that into perspective, when we do massive cancer surgery, we never quote death rates above ten percent. This virus is scary, make no mistakes. It lands you in the wilderness, the worst I have ever experienced; the Lenten experience, (namely praying and fasting) you don't want, but that is thrust upon one.

In all of this though happily for me came a number of angelic presences in the form of some really caring nurses and doctors; people of great empathy and understanding of the physical and psychological tortures of their patients, all living with the high risk of contracting the virus for themselves. I had started with Augmentin and doxycycline as antibiotics, but after a terrible weekend of clearly making no progress, on the Monday morning a dynamic consultant and his excellent team entered my room. He asked a few questions, examined me and commenced a number of changes, probably most significant was the introduction of intravenous Tazocin. I was also sneakily taking my own 'sweeties' in the form of hydroxychloroquine, supplied by a GP friend, now for the record on the Royal Brompton COVID-19 protocol. I received much skilful care from these attendants as well as so many messages of love, support and prayers and friendship from family and friends and thanks to all of this I believe I came to deliverance back to my children and home.

I arrived home half dead, but at least alive, and improving daily. I have two trips planned for later in the year, one to the Isle of Revelation, Patmos, the other to Palestine. Where, ironically, the plan is to venture into the desert where Christ spent his 40 tumultuous days. Fifteen days in the Coronavirus desert proved more than enough for this man.

I will finish with a quote from the great Greek man of letters George Seferis:

'The day before, a little after midnight, "I was in the Isle which is called Patmos." As dawn was breaking, I was in Chora. The sea was motionless and like metal bound the islands around. Not even a leaf

breathed in the strengthening light. The peace was a shell without
the slightest fracture. I remained transfixed by its influence; then
I felt I was whispering: "Come and see ..."'

COVID-19 came in the first wave with much destruction, lives wrecked, and people losing loved ones. Then there was the second wave and lockdown #2. Although this is now much disputed, I, for one, reckon the first two lockdowns saved a lot of lives. In addition, lockdown #3 on the continent seemed justified there, but in my opinion was correctly avoided in the UK. Ironically, Boris called it well, but should never have lied about his partying! I suspect the public might have forgiven the truth, who knows?

These waves of COVID-19 meant the chance of the programme restarting in 2020 or 2021 were nil. However, in 2022, things surgically were returning to normal, and after much effort our deceased programme resumed later in the year. A first living-donor case was planned for early 2023. This will all be described over the next two chapters.

The Patient Journey

Most of the women who wish to have a uterus transplant have in fact been born without one; they have ovaries and a vagina, but sadly, no cervix and/or womb. This is a terrible place to find oneself. The classic story, in the case of MRKH, is of the girl who goes through puberty, but gets to about age 15 or 16 and still has no periods, though she gets some pre-menstrual type symptoms. She is taken by her mother to the GP; a referral is made to a gynaecologist who organises an ultrasound, and then makes the awful discovery of that the patient has no womb. Devastating news, and not something you can talk to your friends about very readily.

In our womb-transplant programme, we also have another group of women who still have a uterus, but it is not functional. Some of these women, though currently on our lists for uterine transplantation, might have a much smaller procedure in the future in the form of endometrial transplantation or new endometrium engineered using stem cells. This was described previously in Chapters 5 and 6. In addition, there are women whose wombs are so damaged by other benign conditions, e.g., fibroids, as to be incapable of reproduction.

Over 1,000 women have approached us seeking womb transplantation, and more than 500 women have contacted us to enquire about donating their uterus. We have met with many of these women; following a detailed pre-screening process, around 20 donors have been investigated and counselled comprehensively. The first patients have been selected for the 10 deceased-donor cases. Those women selected were all required to have five embryos in cold storage. The embryos have all undergone preimplantation genetic testing to maximise the chance of success. The women were then on call until a suitable matched donor organ became available – in the Southeast of England, we believe this occurred at a rate of one per month. This follows the stringent criteria for deceased-organ donation. The other criteria for organ donation are similar to all solid-organ transplants.

8

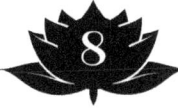

Womb Transplant UK: Deceased Donor Programme — Late 2022

I personally was lying in bed with a slipped disc. Thinking that I was going nowhere and wondering if I was going to have to cancel my Tuesday operating list, my phone pipped with a text from Sal saying there may be a patient suitable for organ donation. At this point I felt extremely apprehensive. There was no way we could turn this down, irrespective of my back. There were texts backwards and forwards throughout the day, and the decision was made to send the scout team once we knew that the blood group worked, the cytomegalo-virus (CMV) status was appropriate and the patient had fulfilled all the criteria. This was a first for our team.

The scout team were mobilised, which included Ben and Sal. They were transported to the hospital where the potential donor was and performed the appropriate tests by way of an infection screen and ultrasound, which showed normal pelvic organs.

We had results by 9ish on Monday morning. I, for one recognised, that I needed to cancel at least some of my clinic and possibly the whole afternoon. Things were duly arranged. It became clear that we were going to meet at 9.15 pm at Queen Charlotte's to go with NHS trans-port back to the site of the donor, and on this occasion the team on the transport were going to be Ben, Sal, and myself, with Srdjan Saso as observer. Isabel and her colleagues were coming on a different transport from Oxford.

It was an interesting evening; I tried to get some sleep between 7 and 8 and somewhat failed because the phone kept going. I had also gone out to purchase a picnic for the team, which came in handy later. I went by taxi to Queen Charlotte's Hospital, where we met with Steve the driver while congregating in a cold carpark. We had a bag of equipment, including McCartney tubes, Ligaclips, spare glasses, clogs etc. We headed off to our destination; I think the team in the back snoozed. I ended up chatting to Steve, and as we arrived in at the retrieval hospital, he showed us all the way to theatres, rang the doorbell and brought us in. Not long after that, Isabel and her colleague Mr Keno Mentor, Consultant in Transplantation Surgery at Coventry, appeared.

We then went into a side room where we had the pre-operative huddle/multidisciplinary team (MDT) meeting with the small-bowel team. The cardiac team were in theatre, and we checked all the consent forms and saw the paperwork, which showed the patient was negative for HPV negative and other screened infections, and also that she had had a negative pregnancy test. We then went round to the operating theatre to have a huddle with the cardiac surgeons and to perform the next pre-operative checklist.

To me, this was a moving event. There were somewhere in the region of 12 surgeons in theatre: our team amounted to four, plus Isabel's colleague, plus two cardiac surgeons, plus the four people from small-bowel team, plus the resident nursing staff and senior nurse from the local hospital, plus Isabel's scrub team and the cardiac scrub team and perfusionist; we also had our own perfusionist. The specialist nurse in organ donation (SNOD) ran this with great skill. There was a minute's silence, which I thought was extremely appropriate and certainly made me reflect on the enormous nature of the evening.

The dissection involved the juxtaposition of skills between Isabel and myself, ably assisted by Ben and Sal, with Srdjan looking on from behind. My whole training is about removing organs with a margin and minimising blood loss, and this means I have a great love of devices and methods like LigaSure, diathermy, etc. Transplant surgeons' eyes are much more focussed on preserving vessels. In fact, many of the predictions we made about the timing of retrievals had been based around oncological procedures where the aforementioned electrical devices were in use. The devices proved not to be totally appropriate on the day, but still somewhat appropriate, and it is fascinating to me that Isabel and I were able to operate backwards and forwards across the table, both, to a degree, modifying our style of surgery. Isabel moved into using the LigaSure, and I certainly moved into realising I had better not LigaSure quite as liberally, as Isabel pointed out that was not the right thing to do in some situations.

At the end of the procedure, we appeared to have obtained a very fine graft indeed. Following the procedure, the last rites were performed. I do know that I stood really struggling to get my head around the enormity of the evening. I personally had not seen anything like this in my life before, and was acutely aware the patient and her family had effectively saved six lives – a lung to one person, a heart to another, a pancreas to another, a liver to another, and the kidneys going in two directions – and additionally had potentially teed up to create a new life with the uterine transplant. This is quite an astonishing thing to do.

As a side note, this came up at the debrief meeting later organised by NHS Blood and Transplant, where the question was asked: 'Who was holding the scissors?' The genuine answer was that it was Isabel and myself, not one person dominating this procedure in any way. In terms of theatre psychology, Isabel certainly was the dominant person in our team, and rightly, so as the lead transplant surgeon. We gynae-cologists all quietly commented at the time that in the new, totally alien environment, without Isabel we would have been sunk without trace.

Srdjan kindly said that he thought we had done the best op he had ever seen. I cannot comment on that but I think my only thought at the time was that this was a totally joint procedure with Isabel, and that is what came home to me on that evening as one of the great strengths of the team. A very good complimentary set of skills and no egos across the table. A rare combination.

We emerged into the carpark to the best Christmas decorations any of us had ever seen in any hospital. We then headed off again, with Steve, the driver for Oxford, fully believing we were about to transplant a uterus. This journey afforded us all an opportunity for a little sleep. It was always accepted that may not deliver a decent graft in the first retrieval we, but it turned out that we appeared to have delivered an excellent graft on every level, and there had been minimal blood loss from our end during the procedure.

We arrived in Oxford; Ben, Sal, Srdjan and myself went to the ward to see the patient, who we knew well. It was a somewhat emotional and almost tearful event, since it is true to say that none of us – the patient, her husband and the surgical team – could actually believe that we were there about to do this. It was really rather surreal. I said we had a little back-table work (which involves preparing the graft for implantation and assessing its vessels) to do, but we expected to send for her in half an hour to an hour to implant the uterus. We went down to theatre to join Isabel at the back-table work. It had been agreed that her back-table work was best done in Oxford, and the cannulation took place showing excellent ovarian vessels; perfect internal iliac veins, a perfect internal iliac artery on the left; and cannulation with good flow. Then unfortunately we came to the right internal iliac and were unable to cannulate the uterine artery. This internal iliac was opened and again the openings (ostia) were narrow – it was cannulatable but nothing perfused. It was then dilated and still nothing perfused. After much discussion it was decided the procedure had to be abandoned.

Afterward, Ben spoke to Liza Johannessen in Dallas, who agreed that we absolutely made the right decision. Interestingly, I spoke to a couple of people the following week, who both said 'why couldn't you have taken vessels from somewhere else?' This is to misunderstand the nature of uterine arteries, which are coiled like a telephone wire and are essential to this procedure; we also know that we need at least two supplying vessels.

Isabel and I went to the ward to see the patient and her partner. Isabel handled this with great care and skill; this was a very emotional meeting. Personally, I shed a tear — we all did. The patient knew she was back on our list and she now, at least, knew that this was for real, and she would likely have a uterine transplant in the next few months.

The following week was one of great reflection; we had come so close but not quite there. At the highly formalised NHSBT debrief meeting, already alluded to above, it transpired that the multi-organ retrieval we undertook on Monday night was one of the largest retrievals ever planned in British transplant history. The meeting became quite emotional on a couple of occasions, not least when the letter was read out from the family about their feelings about the fact that their nearest and dearest had donated not only all of her other organs, but also her uterus. Even though it had transpired not to be a viable graft, they were in no doubt that they had done the right thing, and they wished our team all the very best with our future transplants and hoped that the lessons we learned were beneficial. This almost reduced the entire committee to tears, I have to say.

Over the next few months, we had a number of calls regarding possible donors, but it wasn't until about a year later that a further suitable donor became available for the recipient. I will not describe this in detail, since the procedures were of course very similar. Suffice to say that we had improved our choreography of which surgeons did which bits to afford more rest time, particularly for Isabel, who in the first living-donor case described below was at the table for an inhuman amount of time. It is enough to say that after a year-long wait our recipient received a uterus, made an excellent post-operative recovery, and now menstruates monthly. She is likely to have an embryo transferred into her new womb in the near future.

In February of 2024, a further suitable uterus became available for the woman who had been longest on our list. Happily, she had a successful transplant and is also menstruating monthly.

In the May of 2024, another suitable uterus became available and a successful deceased donor transplant was performed. The patient is now menstruating monthly following her procedure.

Finally, it's important to understand that womb donation is not covered by the NHS Organ Donor Register or the Organ Donation (Deemed Consent) Act 2019, which implemented an opt-out system in the UK. This means that even if someone is an organ donor, their womb cannot be donated unless their family gives additional specific permission after death, and the donation only goes ahead if the family agrees. We, along with the recipients and their families, are all incredibly grateful to those donors who have given their wombs and to their families for their agreement.

Chapter

9

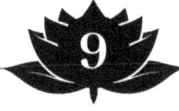

Womb Transplant UK: Living Donor Programme — Early 2023

O n the Friday I had a very light pre-dinner drink with my great friend Rev Gary Bradley and friends at the vicarage, and met my daughter Lara for dinner in a Turkish restaurant in St John's Wood. I was home in reasonably good time for a big night's sleep in anticipation of the events of the weekend. Come Saturday, I had finished my packing and headed for Oxford arriving at approximately 4 pm, where I checked into our hotel. I introduced some organisation into my room, setting it up to work through the week. I was getting ready to walk into Oxford when Isabel texted to say she would pick me up, and we went to mass at the Oxford Oratory — St Aloysius Church, which proved an appropriate start to the events of the weekend. There was a young Irish priest who preached a good sermon, and this certainly got us into the right frame of mind. Isabel dropped me back to the hotel, and I had made an arrangement to eat in the restaurant opposite called Gees. A very charming maitre d' from Sicily greeted me and told me there were no table seats, but I happily agreed to sit at the bar.

This place was important to me, since eight years earlier I had been in this restaurant with Peter Friend, in the company of Stephen Kennedy, to push this project forward in Oxford. It was an amazing thing, then, to sit at the bar in the same restaurant where the whole project had been created. I had a lovely meal of Orkney scallops served in a scallop shell followed by excellent duck ragu. In honour of Isabel and the Spanish connection with this project, which includes Cesar and Paco, I had a very fine carafe of Spanish Rioja. My plan had been that Ben and Sal would turn up probably when I was about two-thirds of the way through this carafe, which is what duly happened. Ben and I shared the end of it, meaning there was no excess of alcohol on the night before the unfolding process.

I was up at 6.15 am and we all met outside. I had the car ready with the SatNav on to take us to the Churchill Transplant Centre, leaving at 6.45 and arriving at 7. This all worked like clockwork, and between 7 and 8, all the various members of the team arrived. From the London end, the complete group consisted of myself, Ben, Sal, Srdjan Saso, and Cesar Diaz-Garcia, all with consultant contracts. Srdjan, in fact, had only obtained his Oxford contract that Friday. Ahmad Sayasneh was also there as an observer.

At the Oxford end, there were a huge number of staff who had given freely of their time and effort. These included the Senior Theatre

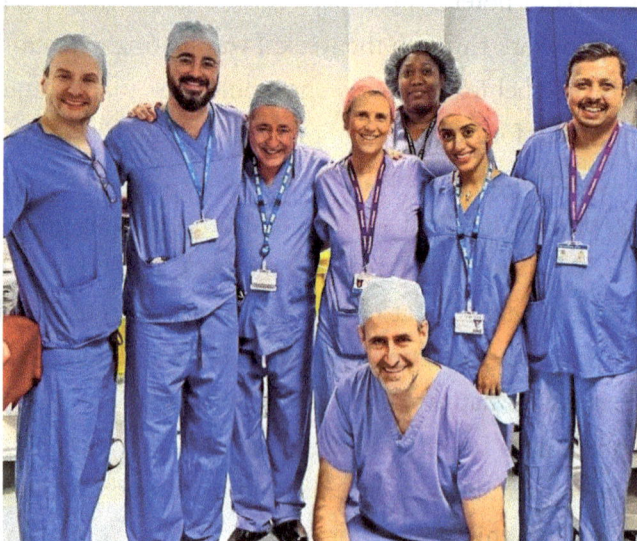

Core surgical team (left to right): Srdjan, Ben, Richard, Isabel, Ann (behind), Cesar (in front), Sal, Venkatesha.

Sister Jo Nawrocka for the retrieval process, plus many nurses and other staff as acknowledged on page xviii. In this process, a remarkable man, Antonio Barbosa, was prepared to switch his cell saver for collecting and recirculating blood at 9.30 am on the Sunday morning. He did not finally switch it off till 5.30 am on Monday morning.

There were three brilliant anaesthetists — Drs Peter Dimitrov, Richard Katz and Andris Klucniks. There was a lot of enthusiasm in the room, and all of us had brought food. Dr Dimitov's wife, Dr Lucy Cogwell, had baked a cake; Sal had brought a home-made cake; Isabel had been to the supermarket and ordered vast amounts of food, and in fact had been given extra free food. The managers Yassmin and Bryony came to wish us luck and brought home-made cakes and brownies. I turned up with the smelliest cheese in the world, which smelt like a farmyard but actually tasted amazing, along with my usual Mediterranean stuff. There were huge quantities of soft drinks. Most of this had been consumed by the following morning.

We then commenced with a huddle, where approximately 30 people introduced themselves, and said where they were from; this was followed by a breakfast. I had given Isabel the cold meats I had brought along, and she had taken these home to her fridge. The rest of my stuff remained in the car boot, probably contributing to the odour from the cheese! This allowed me to have what I personally need before any major op, which is some sort of bacon and carbohydrate, so I had salami and croissants and felt much better. I had a single coffee and no shaky hands, and at 9.50 am we had the donor on the table.

We opened the abdomen, and interestingly, after all the stuff that we had debated in Dallas in 2019 about using a large vertical scar or a cosmetically-more-acceptable low horizontal scar, we had finally alighted on the latter, a Maylard incision (one that does involve muscle-cutting, not as bad as it sounds). We had spoken with Isabel on a WhatsApp call two weeks earlier at Hammersmith, and she agreed that the exposure was brilliant, and so 'Maylard incision it was.' We opened the abdomen, stitched the peritoneum back, and the major dissection ensued, resulting in the retrieval of the uterus, cervix, parametrium, uterosacral and round ligaments, plus a substantial piece of anterior peritoneum from across the bladder.

This process, somewhat like the previous explant, involved the backwards and forwards across the table between Isabel and myself. It is disturbing after 40 years of surgery and 30 years as a consultant oncological surgeon to discover that one's skill mix is not quite adequate for the purpose of transplantation; this is undoubtedly different whereby vessels must be preserved at all costs and not damaged by any of the thermal devices that we love to use. Also, a gentle approach to tissue, very important in cancer surgery, turned out to be even more so in the transplant context. We were slightly thrown by some quite unusual anatomy in the vascular structures, whereby the anterior division of the internal iliac on the right gave off, within the space of a centimetre, two uterine arteries (two uterine arteries are very rare), the superior vesical artery, and the obliterated hypogastric.

The notes from Dallas in 2019 proved invaluable with respect to double-slinging the ureters and using the inferior hypogastric as our vessel to tract on. Double-slinging involves putting a sling around the ureter on either side of the uterine arteries and veins. This allowed very rapid access to double-slinging of the ureter on the left side. On the right side, though, I thought I might have placed the sling around the ureter but did not feel confident about this at all. After some discussion, it was decided we should stent the left ureter. Cesar had told us earlier that within the Swedish series, the ureters were always stented beforehand, and this is a path we will follow from now on in living donors.

There is a lot of stress involved with stenting ureters mid-operation, since there is a small chance that one will fail to insert the stent, at which point one's back is seriously against the wall. Happily, this did not happen. The first stent went up easily; the second stent proved more difficult and in fact there was a little cheer as I duly inserted the catheter. These came out at the end of the operation, and as always, they caused haematuria (blood in the urine). Having now gotten firm ureteric identification, it became much easier to dissect the entire arterial venous plexus in a safe fashion. Cesar later commented we should have done more lateral pelvic sidewall dissection, and I agree with this. One of the issues on this particular day was that there was a vast number of people, as this was the first time this operation had been performed in the UK. The Imperial team had not operated before in Oxford, and I will confess to having had some anxieties that morning. As a surgeon in the operating theatre, it is vital to maintain the confidence of all the staff, both medical and nursing. This is even more acute when you are in a new environment. I was apprehensive about any chance of a major bleed early on, something which rarely happens but can happen on the lateral pelvic sidewall, hence my slightly more timid approach at this point. The prospect of disaster loomed heavily, particularly upon Isabel and myself. In future, we will take the bolder approach down the pelvic sidewalls earlier on than we did.

At the point where we had decent mobilisation incorporating the structures as detailed above, a wet swab was placed over the abdomen, and we departed for a late lunch. At this point, it was 3.30 or 4.00 in the afternoon. We came back from a brief lunch and completed the dissection with retrieval of the uterus and surrounding structures, which then went to the back table, as per the plan. Isabel, Ben and Ann went to the back table. Approximately an hour before the retrieval was complete, Venkatesha and Srdjan had gone to the next theatre to open the recipient, and they had laid bare the external iliac vessels and commenced preparation for the implantation.

Whilst the back-table work was going on, Cesar and Sal and I completed the procedure on the donor. We completed the operation pretty much in sync with Isabel finishing the back-table work, which had proved taxing. Professor Peter Friend and Mr Sanjay Sinha had both been to the theatre to see how we were doing and wish us well; the overwhelming feeling of support from the Churchill transplant staff was quite astonishing. This was a difficult day, and we thought we were well through it, but we were a long way off still.

The uterus was then taken through to Theatre 8; it was of particular importance to me that we were using Theatre 7 and 8, since these are the numbers on the Theatres that we use at Hammersmith. In these circumstances, one is always looking for familiarity. For the record, I am also very superstitious; no patient gets 13 clips, and synchronous theatre numbers induce a feel-good factor – not too scientific, I'll grant you.

The uterus was then placed within the abdomen and the vessel hook-up proceeded. This was primarily done by Isabel, Venkatesha, Ann and Ben, with the rest of us coming in and out to observe. Having laid the uterus into the abdomen, it became clear it was important to remove the uterine remnants prior to the anastomoses. Interestingly, these remnants incorporated small 3 × 2 cm tubular structures on each side with normal Fallopian tubes, with a stretch of uterine tissue going across between them. There was also what felt like a residuum of cervix. I therefore removed the Fallopian tubes and the uterine remnants and mobilised the bladder. We inserted methylene blue into the bladder to aid its identification; we were well clear on this aspect of the dissection, and removed most of the tissue, leaving what was effectively a vestige of what might have been cervix. This proved to be extremely useful later as a support structure, which we utilised along with the uterosacral ligaments (a band of tissue connecting the uterus to the base of the spine). The uterosacral ligaments were separately clamped and ligated with a tie put on. This was later stitched onto the remnant, which itself was stitched on to the vagina, thus providing excellent uterine support along with the round ligaments and peritoneum.

Having performed what was effectively a sub-total removal of uterine remnants, I handed the reins back to the transplant team. The anastomoses went forward with the help of very skilful microvascular surgery performed by Isabel and Venkatesha, and not helped by the patient's strange anatomy, with two uterine vessels per side. Once the vessels were complete, the gynaecological structures, ligaments, and peritoneum (the membrane surrounding the abdominal organs)

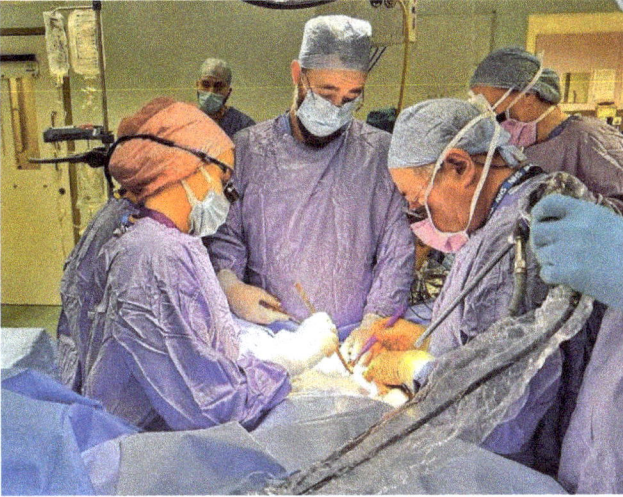

The team transplanting. From left to right: Isabel, Antonio (background), Ben, Richard, Srjdan (background).

were sutured in. The vaginal anastomoses was performed using lubricated interrupted sutures. Again, Cesar provided great reassurance and knowledge from the original Swedish transplant programme. By the end of this process, we had appropriate arterial and venous connections, and had achieved a good set-up regarding uterine support.

There was much debate about inserting a Doppler device to measure blood flow. We made the decision to do so; the device was placed round the uterine vessels and made this wonderful Doppler whooshing noise, which demonstrated that our graft had a good blood supply. Cesar declared our graft to be good, and that, along with the whooshing noise, made us all very happy. The abdomen was closed in standard fashion.

By this time, it was 5.30 am, with a very exhausted but happy team. We took team photos, and I made a very short vote of thanks, basically to thank everybody for their unbelievable effort over what was now a 21- or 22-hour period. The patient went to recovery, and we came back to the hotel. It should be noted that we had regularly phoned the family of the two sisters throughout this long day of huge stress for all of them.

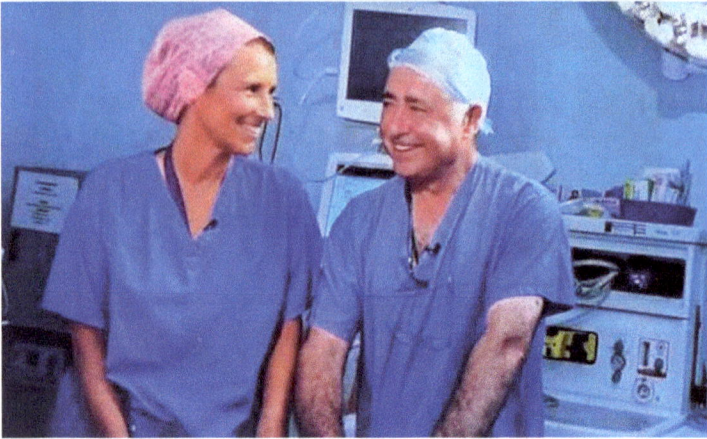

Isabel and Richard, happy with the outcome!

I have no idea how Isabel kept going with 21 hours of surgery, since I was exhausted after having done nine hours and then two or three more. As I noted earlier, we changed the surgeon's choreography going forward to prevent this from happening again. Ben, Sal, Cesar and I had a glass of champagne at 6.30 that morning in my room. I put the bottle in the car, thinking along the Lillie Bollinger quote, 'I drink Champagne when I'm happy and when I'm sad ...'. We might have something to celebrate, and if we don't, we will have something to feel sorry about. Happily, it was the former. We drank the champagne pretty rapidly. There was some thumping on the ceiling and wall of my room from neighbours who were probably thinking 'drunk students' — drunk, no, students, yes.

There is no doubting that this was the most unbelievable day I personally have ever experienced as a surgeon. The explant six weeks prior was another unbelievable day, and it took me back to when we first did the abdominal radical trachelectomy and modified Strassman procedures. These are amazing learning experiences full of stress and worry, and always, 'Please, God let it be okay for our patients.'

The following day the donor looked to be in very good health, recovering as one would expect from what is in essence a modified radical hysterectomy. The recipient also looked to be in excellent health. The husbands of the two women and their parents must have had unbelievable anxieties, notwithstanding our phone calls of reassurance. They are a delightful family, and we have all desperately wanted to help them – and please, God, I hope that we have. This project had been criticised from the outset for, among other things, creating unreasonable expectations, so the stakes were high.

One of the hard things in post-operative care is that after a cancer operation, you kind of know if all is well in the first 24 to 48 hours. That applied here to the donor, but when it comes to the recipient, it was a whole new world of transplantation surgery, which us gynaecologists are not really familiar with. It had all been theoretical until then; now it was for real, and wow, is it anxiety-creating. I had no idea how Isabel had coped with the previous day's length of surgery; I personally was wrecked after what I did, and Isabel was effectively operating for an extra 10 hours over and above me – a remarkable and astonishing achievement. Also, when it comes to the entirety of the staff of the Churchill Transplant Centre, they again made a stellar performance.

Looking back over the week, as Cesar told us, it was 10 years to the exact weekend that the Swedes first transplanted a uterus, and for me personally, it had been 25 years since I transplanted a uterus in a porcine model and seven and a half years since we originally obtained Ethics Committee approval to perform this procedure. Sam Abdalla and I had met in 1996 after an abdominal radical trachelectomy at the Rising Sun near the Lister Hospital. When we talked for the first time about uterine transplant, I had asked Sam, "How many people were out there who needed this procedure?" He replied that it was up to 10% of infertility patients. This had been some journey.

Things progressed reasonably smoothly until mid-week. Isabel had gone home for dinner and Sal was in town meeting friends. I was feeling quite relaxed, having booked into the restaurant at the hotel and had one course of fish and chips, when suddenly a flurry of texts came through: the recipient was bleeding, and the much-previously-loved probe was giving a weak signal. Sal and I spoke; she was coming back in a taxi, so I jumped in her taxi as it passed our hotel on the way to the Churchill Transplant Centre.

We were there for a couple of hours. An ultrasound showed good myometrial blood flow and the Doppler imaging to the vessels was perfect. Ben had phoned Liza Johannesson and she had reassured us that the Doppler probe's signal would get weaker if there was fluid around it. In fact it, transpired the patient was over-heparinised (heparin is a blood thinning medication used to prevent blood clots). We had a discussion with Isabel and a new regime was introduced. Isabel's motto is: 'We'd much rather a bleed, because we can stop that, than a clot because we can do nothing about that – and we do not want a thrombosed organ, that's when it's all over!' As cancer surgeons, we hate bleeding. The next decision was whether to transfuse blood. It is interesting that the transplant people do not like transfusing until the haemoglobin is down to 7 grams per decilitre because of issues with potential antibodies, but here we were in a situation where some blood was required, I suggested 3 to 4 units; Isabel said 1, maybe 2, and to reduce the heparin; she turned out to be right.

The following day we then went over to the Churchill Transplant Centre, and our two patients were both looking excellent. I had always envisaged that I might slip out of Oxford for a walk in the country, but I didn't dare to. The following day, the now-dreaded Doppler dislodged, creating more anxieties, but a further scan confirmed normality in the graft.

The following day, Isabel phoned me to say that the recipient was losing lymphatic fluid from her vagina; this time, I was able to say 'we don't worry about that at all.' Loss of lymphatic fluid is completely standard after removing pelvic lymph nodes, which of course we did when preparing the vessels. This, again, is an indicator of the combined skills of the team, and of good communication. Isabel, Sal and I had a great meeting later in the day where we planned a charity dinner to get everybody from Oxford and London into one room for a huge 'thank-you.' (This dinner happened four months later, raising £70,000.) The three of us returned to Gees for dinner that night for what was effectively a counselling session for post-traumatic stress disorder (PTSD).

The following day, it was planned that we would take the first biopsy to check for rejection. This was to be performed in theatre without anaesthesia. Isabel was comfortable that Sal and I were heading back to London with the histopathology samples from the cervix but Sal would return on Saturday to see the patients, and I personally would be back on Sunday to the same end.

The minor biopsy procedure without anaesthetic utilised a colposcope — a microscope used to visualise the cervix. We were able to see quite a normal-looking cervix, pink in colour, which when biopsied bled in an appropriately minor way which we stopped. Biopsies were taken at the 12 and 6 o'clock positions. There are no functional nerve endings in the cervix in the initial post-transplant phase, so there was no pain associated with the biopsies. We then came to realise that whilst we had some arrangements in place, our expected histopathologist was unfortunately on holiday. We had to pull in a big favour from the non-immunological but gynaecological histopathologist Dr Baljeet Kaur. Baljeet went the distance for us, phoning Dr Andrew Gallimore, Laboratory Director, who was in South Africa, to get permission to perform the analysis. The donor was discharged home that day.

By six o'clock that evening we had the views of both Baljeet and the pathologist at the Baylor University Medical Center (Dallas), which agreed that our biopsy was perfect, and showed no signs of rejection. This was great news. One of the amazing things about the whole week was how many people bent over backwards to make things happen. The radiologists the morning prior, after the recipient was wheeled out of the theatre back to the ward, said to bring the patient so that we would all know that the flows were fine. The recipient was discharged home soon thereafter.

That week proved the most stressful of my career, and I think the same can be said for Isabel, Ben and Sal. We knew from the world literature that at the point where the uterus is implanted, there is a 20% chance of it requiring removal. By the time we had a normal biopsy five days later, this chance had probably dropped to 5%. Imagine our joy when, a week later, we had a further normal biopsy taken by Ben, and the patient had her first menstrual period post-transplant. The data has shown that the vast majority of women who menstruate post-transplant go on to have a baby. To paraphrase Winston Churchill, 'never, in the field of gynaecology, was a period so much desired by so many for one woman.' Ben and I were dining together that evening, and on receiving the results, phoned Isabel and Sal, and texted the extended team; finally, we felt that we could all relax a bit, and Ben and I had a little celebration.

Twelve months later the donor and recipient are well, with the recipient menstruating monthly from her new womb, which is normal on scanning. The two women and their families had gone through a huge event while demonstrating good humour and great understanding. The extended Oxford team were stellar, the nursing and anaesthetic teams were just amazing, and the whole thing truly humbling. Since then, Isabel, Ben, Andrea Devaney, Claire Snelgrove, Katie Jeffery and Sal have done much ongoing work to keep our patients safe, in particular to maintain appropriate levels of immunosuppression. Across our patients, a number of embryo transfers have now taken place.

Returning to our overall programme, when the women are called for deceased or living donor transplant, they go to Oxford to receive their new uterus. Their care is then undertaken between Oxford and London, and it is intensive. After a minimum of six months, embryo transfer takes place at the Lister Hospital, with one embryo being transferred at a time to minimise the risk of twin pregnancy.

Once pregnant, they are looked after in early pregnancy by Miss Maya Al-Memar and in later pregnancy by Miss Bryony Jones both at Queen Charlotte's and Chelsea Hospital, where their delivery will be made by Caesarean section. Three to six months later, they can have a completion hysterectomy or try for another baby. If they have a second child, the uterus will be removed three to six months after the birth. They can then stop their immunosuppressive therapy. This relatively short exposure of two to five years minimises the risks of long-term immunosuppressive therapy, namely cancer and infection. There has been much speculation as to whether the completion hysterectomy could be avoided by just stopping the immunosuppressive therapy, and the uterus could just wither away. However, this may result in the recipient developing antibodies, which may be problematic in the future in the case that they may require a blood transfusion or another organ transplant.

Another suggestion has been made that at completion hysterectomy the uterus could be used again in another recipient. Again, this resides in the arena of theory, and in truth, due to the small vessel size, I believe it is unlikely to happen.

Chapter

10

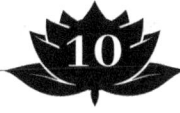

Personal Reflections
from the Team

Miss Isabel Quiroga-Giraldez

At the time of writing, I am 10 years into this collaboration with my Imperial College gynaecological colleagues. This section is divided into two parts, the first dealing with the science from a transplant perspective and the latter more with my journey emotionally on this project — including being a surgeon and a mother, not an easy combination. It's been quite a journey, but it now very much feels like a relationship of equals.

I was asked if I would like to help colleagues from London develop their deceased-donor retrieval techniques and facilitate the integration of the gynaecology team into the multi-organ abdominal retrieval process. As the clinical lead for Organ Retrieval in Oxford, I was well-situated to offer my advice. I will confess to having had some serious reservations as to the wisdom of the whole project. I felt quite uncertain as to whether these gynaecologists, with their cancer and infertility backgrounds, really understood the risks associated with transplant surgery. I also worried that the patients had little idea as to the risks they might encounter.

In 2014, I invited the gynaecology team to the National Organ Retrieval master class that my colleague Rutger Ploeg and I organised. I thought this would be the perfect induction to the donation and

retrieval process. It would also deliver the necessary NHSBT certifi-
cation to join the National Organ Retrieval Service. This was the first
time I met Richard and his colleagues face-to-face. and I was reassured
that this was a group of surgeons who I could work with.

In 2015, I attended Womb Transplant UK's first charity dinner at
the House of Lords, which proved pivotal to my thinking. I met and
listened to a patient who had gone down the route of surrogacy in order
to have a family. That meeting and her speech convinced me that to
help women with no functional womb to carry their own babies must
be right for at least some of them.

Originally, the team planned only to go down the route of deceased
donors, although that expanded to dual living- and deceased-donor
programmes in 2019. It had been demonstrated that a new technique,
developed by the Dallas team, had greatly shortened the donor operation, thus improving safety for the patient. Adding living donors also
entailed a new layer of regulation.

Since then, we have developed a real partnership across the gynaecology, transplant, IVF and obstetrics fields. My own background is in
kidney and pancreatic transplantation; early on, colleagues said to me
that kidney transplant and uterine transplant are technically similar. In
2016, I went to Gothenburg for a master class, with the words ringing
in my ears: 'the uterine vessels are just like a living-donor kidney transplant,' the latter being an operation I do very frequently. I saw videos
and was not convinced. Then in 2019, at the National Retrieval master
class in Bristol, I saw those tiny uterine vessels. Admittedly this was in
an old cadaver; the vessels are bigger in a young woman, but they are
still tiny compared to renal vessels. The uterine and ovarian veins bear
no resemblance to renal veins. This means we have had to think long
and hard about those technical aspects, and creating an appropriate
number of arterial and venous anastomoses, to ensure graft viability.

One of the things I realised early on in this programme was the
importance of becoming more than merely a surgical technician. My
understanding of transplant surgery and medicine were all coming into

play with that of my gynaecological colleagues, and that we both had much to contribute, from our very different standpoints, to the overall care of the patients.

The understanding of transplant is difficult, and after long years you develop a sixth sense as to where trouble looms. The difficulty with uterine transplant is that these women are healthy – the direct opposite of those with kidney failure or diabetes. All transplant patients have to comply with their medication, or their graft will fail. Our uterine transplant patients are not used to taking medication and don't know what it is like to feel and be ill. The risk is there, however, of potential rapid deterioration surgically and medically, including risks of opportunistic infection and cancer. The patients need multiple assessments – gynaecological, transplant, psychological – as well as anaesthetic review. We originally thought to keep hospital visits to a minimum before the transplant, but experience has now taught us that this is the wrong approach. Patients need time to assimilate the information, balance the risks, and come to the right decision for them and their families. Our specialist nurse, Clare Snelgrove, has been pivotal in this process, supporting patients who are navigating this process.

We rapidly discovered that post-operative follow-up needs to be shared between the two groups, both of whom have their own slightly differing anxieties. It is essential that one member of the gynaecology team remain in Oxford post-op, and essential that on the longer-term follow up the patients are seen both at Oxford and at Imperial, to maximise input from both groups. There are variations between laboratories in different hospitals with regards to virological monitoring, a classic example, with Imperial and Oxford using differing techniques that are not 100% transferrable. We originally thought that remote management might be possible, but it has proved vitally important that the patients attend both institutions, to benefit from the differing skill sets of the transplant surgery and gynaecology teams.

I now want to move to the story that forms the backdrop behind the science. The first thing was the risk for our whole project if we had failed in the first living or deceased donor cases; there is no doubt in my mind that failure in either of those cases would have resulted in the closure of both the living and deceased projects. All the systems that are in place across the health service are risk-averse, and while on one level that is great and appropriate, on another, it makes major innovation very difficult and personally risky. It is, of course, totally correct that the regulatory structure is as robust as it is. Transplantation surgery is rightly one of the most highly-regulated areas in medicine in the UK.

Over these years, the Oxford Transplant Centre has had a number of managers that have delivered different levels of support for the project. However, our most recent managers – Bryony Lennon, Senior Operations Manager, Yassmin Khater, Service Manager, and Rebecca Cullen, Service Manager – have proven to be a tower of support. They have been instrumental because they totally believe in the project. When these three women came along, it was a total transformation. They were going to make it happen! Rebecca did extensive training, dedicating hours of her own time to become an HTA Independent Assessor. Bryony and Yassmin were so excited the week of the transplant; that's when they felt they wanted to come with us. They turned up at 7.30 am that first Sunday morning, having baked the most delicious brownies, just to wish us luck. I was deeply touched and delighted that they wanted to feel part of the whole thing, and the fact that they were there was amazing. I was really proud that they got there. Andrea Devaney has also supported the project over five years with protocol writing, patient care and more.

The other aspect was our senior nursing staff, who were so supportive, and Sister Lee was instrumental. She had been a Senior Sister previously at the Churchill Hospital, and we always worked very well together. She spent some time elsewhere, but very happily for our project, she arrived back with us as a Deputy Matron. She just took the uterus transplant programme on board and made it happen. Sister Lee and her colleagues worked extremely hard to make the logistics in the theatre department work at the operational level. Without all these wonderful nursing and managerial friends, the uterus transplant would never have happened.

I knew we needed to have a strong team around us on the day. I have worked for years with a group of dedicated and extremely skilful theatre nurses, whom I trust and respect. I believe that feeling is mutual. I approached every single theatre nurse personally, and everyone was so excited to take part.

My transplant anaesthetic colleagues, Drs Peter Dimitrov and Andris Klucniks, have been on board from day one. They generously assess patients in their free time, and have championed the project to other colleagues. Their professionalism and patient care are legendary, and I was certain that they were best-placed to look after our patients. Dr Richard Katz joined the anaesthetic team later, and has proven to be a wonderful choice.

A consultant surgeon leading a team always needs colleagues they know are totally supportive, with complementary skills, operating with trust and confidence in each other, thus creating an environment allowing one to perform highly complex surgery. I feel blessed to have had Venkatesha and Ann as such colleagues, supporting me in theatre and throughout the tortuous post-operative care of these women.

Returning to the surgery, we were truly blessed that all ended well with the surgery in the first few cases. If we had had problems later on, we might have been forgiven, but not at the start, because they would have been directly attributed to the operation and our surgery. On the day of the first transplant, as you can imagine, the pressure I felt was immense. I know Richard was in the same boat. Here were two of us, risking our reputations on two operations, living donor hysterectomy and transplant, that we had practised as much as we could in a labora-tory setting – but that is never the same as doing it for real.

Now for my very personal feelings on the day. Before the proce-dure, I asked myself if I am the right person to do this. This is a form of imposter syndrome – *are any of my other colleagues better than me?* However, once I am on the ward pre-operatively, my confidence buoys up and I feel certain I can absolutely do the necessary with my team of colleagues.

In that first transplant – both the retrieval and the implantation – all my skills and those of my colleagues across the entire team came together to allow us to succeed in very difficult circumstances. The vessels for anastomosis were smaller and more delicate than first suspected, coupled with some unusual anatomy.

Another aspect that I don't talk a lot about is family life as a mother. You have all these things you need to look after; you want to be a working mother, but also look after your child. For me, for instance, the one bit that defines this conundrum took place the night before the first retrieval – this epitomises my life. I pretend that I am a wonderful mother, the Nigella Lawson, domestic goddess, when I am not any of that, because I want to be this wonderful mother. As a working mother you want to pretend that you can do it all. This idea is 'the big lie,' as my good friend Irene Mosca says.

One story epitomised the BIG LIE concept. I am in the middle of setting up and organising all the logistics for the first ever UK uterine transplant retrieval – phone calls galore, so many decisions, so much uncertainty and second-guessed timings. In the meantime, my son Jaime and I are poorly. I have a temperature and Jaime feels awful, but it's the last week of school before Christmas, he has a Latin exam and we need to revise. I decide that the music teachers are great and Jaime needs to give them a Christmas present – so I am a goddess that can make things and bake and cook. I bought a magazine, and the pictures of marshmallow dips looked amazing. So I make everything; I have a lovely Christmas tin to put everything in, but some jars will not fit the other tin. Then, my husband comes out with the idea of a shoe box. I spent an hour wrapping it in Christmas paper, rather than just keeping the Nike logo on the front. It looks truly professional, but a bit empty, as it is bigger than I planned.

Then I decide I should make something else. It is now past midnight when I start the chocolate marzipan … keep in mind that throughout all this, I am still sorting the uterine transplant. I should be resting, as I know I will not sleep the following night. I finally went to bed at 2.00 am very pleased with myself.

In the morning, there is total pandemonium, and I need to take Jaime to school and to revise more for the Latin exam. There is a massive rush to leave the house. I then remember I need the cookie dough that we have in our chest freezer for the Christmas sale at the school on Saturday. I need to take it to my friend's house for baking day Tuesday. More drama ensues as I am trying to load Jaime in the car, with his school bag, the trumpet, music bag, the homemade presents, and the cookie dough. My retrieval kit in another bag. I cannot find my handbag, and we cannot unplug the car.

When we arrived at the school, Jaime is in the car with the school bag, the trumpet and the music bag, but the bag with the presents is nowhere to be seen! These teachers are having their wretched presents even if they are allergic to nuts and hate marshmallows! So my husband starts looking for the bag all over the house and after 20 minutes finds it …

I had taken it to the garage, put it on the ground and then … run over it with my car! My precious box was destroyed, but the contents were intact, and the tin was good. So I hope the trumpet teacher has a good sense of humour, because he gets the box that had ended up under the wheels of my car!

This was a fantastic story that all the mothers heard at school. Some didn't understand it at all, and others thought it was the funniest thing they heard that day, especially after a couple of glasses of something. I know I suffer a lot for my work and a lot of what I do is a choice. Do I get involved with new things – do I really want to get involved? Do I want to spend more time working? All of this is extra, it is that much extra, and no one is paying you on top of your normal job, so is this fair on one's family or what?

With respect to my son Jaime, he is quite proud of what we have achieved but it has not always been this way. In truth, he hates my job – he doesn't like it at all. He hates all the nights I'm away and transplant surgery involves a lot of night work.

I have to conclude that overall, it's been a marvellous experience. The joint operating between the two teams has been just great as we have improved our operating room choreography and as trust and confidence have built between us, so I can genuinely say we have gone from two teams to one big team. We also appear to be creating a sustainable programme. There have been and continue to be many stresses and strains, but overall, I feel I have done the right thing to the best of my abilities. I have been amazed at the number of women coming forward to be altruistic donors, and am certain that uterine transplant is the best option for some women. Women make choices and risk their health daily in pursuit of motherhood. We have given the opportunity so far to a few women and the hope of motherhood to many, and that's quite something.

Mr Ben Jones

I joined the team almost 12 years ago, as a fresh-faced PhD student. As a surgically-orientated budding fertility specialist, I found the idea of transplanting a uterus into a woman who did not have one audacious and exciting. It was something I believed would forever change the landscape of reproductive medicine and, more importantly, the lives of countless women around the world. Most of my friends, family and colleagues actually thought it was a ridiculous idea that may not have any impact upon the landscape of reproductive medicine, and may even negatively impact my career, should it not be successful. Though at the time it may have seemed more like science fiction than a feasible medical procedure, I had already made a habit of not doing as I was told, and I wasn't going to stop that now; I was determined to be part of the team to make this happen in the UK.

When I first joined the team, I was tasked with taking the concept from an animal model research concept into a feasible procedure in women to restore their fertility. I spent the first year writing the protocols and ethics applications and liaising with the relevant organisations. Following approval, I screened more than 200 women who wanted to undergo the process and invited the first of them to be comprehensively evaluated to determine their suitability to undergo the process.

This is when I first met the brave women who eventually underwent the first uterus transplant cases in the UK. There were times, when I was discussing the risks of the surgery or immunosuppression, when I would ask myself why these young, fit and healthy women would put themselves at such risk, when they had alternative routes to parenthood like adoption or surrogacy. But despite the enormous list of possible and potentially very serious risks, almost all of these women nodded agreeably, their courage and motivation completely unfazed. Nothing I could say could deter them.

By the time I finished with my PhD, it was the first wave of the COVID-19 pandemic, and we still hadn't done a transplant. While this was highly frustrating, I remained happy we were all still alive! Whilst the aim of my PhD to achieve pregnancies in women after uterus transplantation was not achieved, I did manage to achieve a pregnancy in a woman who did not need one — my wife! By the end of my research time, I was a proud father to two beautiful children; Scarlett and Lucius. I watched with amazement how my wife Claire's tummy grew, I felt my children move and kick, and held them both the moment they were born. Our lives were changed inconceivably forever, with feelings of love and pride that I didn't know were possible. These experiences are etched into my heart, where they will remain eternally, and I now truly understand the value of pregnancy and parenthood — and I was a mere bystander! How foolish I was to doubt the motivations of all the women I had met who were desperate to have the opportunity to experience what I had! The immeasurable emotion and pleasure my children have given me is indescribable and make the complexities and risks of uterine transplantation now appear insignificant by comparison; the women's unfazed, agreeable nods now make so much sense.

Once I became a consultant, I was rewarded with my dream job working as a gynaecologist and fertility specialist at the Lister Fertility Clinic in London. Over the last 10 years, I had had the honour of getting to know the woman who underwent our first case, whom I have been with at every step of the way. Rather fittingly, I was now in a position to do her embryo transfer, the final step of her path to becoming pregnant. Almost 18 months after her operation, I was in a clinic room with her and her partner, just like I was when I met them both ten years previously. In that time, so much had happened; they had travelled the world together, moved house, and changed jobs, but they still had this beautiful enduring vulnerability. Despite the incredible rollercoaster they had been on since the transplant, with sadly more downs than ups, they remained unwavering in their trust in me, the team, and the process. The embryo transfer was very straightforward, almost anticlimactic. Immediately afterward, a strange feeling of positivity came across me, one of overwhelming certainty that she would become pregnant, a sensation I had never felt before. The next nine days were filled with hope and excitement.

The day of the pregnancy test came, and I awoke early, in anticipation for the result. I reached for my phone and saw a message on the screen from her, a crying-faced emoji. My heart skipped a beat and my mouth instantly went dry. I put my phone back down, lay back on my pillow, and took a moment to compose myself before picking it back up again to reply to her. After opening up the message I saw the dreaded crying faced emoji was beneath a photo of a pregnancy test. I looked closer, my eyes still blurry from recently awakening, and saw with amazement as it said 'Pregnant; 1–2 weeks.' The tears from the crying-faced emoji were not of sadness; they were tears of joy! Two weeks later I performed the first scan and showed them their baby for the first time. Three crying-faced emojis would have perfectly described that day — all tears of happiness.

I have no doubts being part of this team will be the best part of my career. Almost 12 years on from joining, I may now not be so fresh-faced, but I have yet again been a bystander watching something truly remarkable unfold. Getting to know these brave women is an honour, and it has been a privilege to help them achieve something that they were always told would not be possible. This is our story of how we performed the first cases in the UK, but the story of uterus transplantation is still being written, and there will hopefully be many more chapters, and many more healthy babies, in the future.

Mr Venkatesha Udupa

Embarking on the journey of being a part of the team starting the uterine transplant programme in the UK has been a deeply personal and professional milestone.

I was humbled when I was asked to join the programme by my transplant consultant surgeon colleague, Miss Isabel Quiroga-Giraldez, a year prior to the COVID-19 pandemic. I am aware of the immense potential it holds – not just for medical advancement, but for transforming the lives of women who have longed for the chance to experience pregnancy and childbirth. This is especially clear to me after hearing stories from my wife, who is a fertility specialist. Even today, she gets good-will messages on a daily basis from her former patients who had children following fertility treatment.

I realise that the road to this point has been long, marked by years of training, research, getting clearance from various regulatory bodies, and the collective effort of a multidisciplinary team from Oxford Transplant Centre and Imperial College London. Getting to know about the many years of research done in the field of uterine transplant by Prof Richard Smith and his team from Imperial College London was a revelation to me.

Uterine transplantation is more than just a surgical procedure; it embodies hope and the fulfilment of dreams that were once thought impossible. The prospect of offering this to women in the UK fills me with a profound sense of purpose. With this excitement comes the responsibility. The careful patient selection, the potential risks and the ethical complexities involved, require a delicate balance of caution and optimism.

I am also aware of the collaborative nature of this endeavour. Success depends not only on surgical precision but also on the support of a diverse team of specialists – gynaecologists, obstetricians, fertility experts, pharmacists, transplant coordinators, anaesthetists, pathologists, and a wide array of nurses, including theatre staff, amongst others.

The planned start of the programme in early 2020 had to be paused due to the COVID-19 pandemic. On 23 February, a Sunday, we started the programme by performing the first living donor uterine transplant. In order to lessen the disruption to other surgical services in the hospital, we chose Sunday as the day for the surgery. One team started off with donor surgery. Towards the end of the donor hysterectomy surgery, the second team started off with the recipient operation in another operation theatre. After readying the uterus for transplantation, my consultant colleague joined me in the recipient surgery. We then worked on joining arteries and veins of the uterus to the recipient's arteries and veins. As the size of the uterine vessels are really small, joining them to recipient vessels was a technical challenge. We had to redo the anastomosis on three of those vessels, as first anastomosis had not been good enough.

Once the blood supply was established, then came the vaginal anastomosis and closure of the abdominal wound. Surgery lasted for more than 12 hours. Our resilience as a team and background as transplant surgeons were crucial in making the surgery a success. Both donor and recipient did well in the post-operative period. Following the initial success, we have done three more uterine transplants, all from deceased donors. All the transplant recipients are now in various stages of fertility treatment. The patients' courage and trust are the driving forces behind our work, and it is our duty to honour that by delivering the best possible outcomes.

Looking ahead, I am filled with a sense of anticipation. The journey will undoubtedly be challenging, with unforeseen obstacles and moments of doubt. Yet, I am committed to this path, driven by the potential to change lives and contribute to the evolving landscape of reproductive medicine.

As I take these first steps, I do so with humility, knowing that the success of this programme will be measured not just by medical achievements, but by the joy and fulfilment it brings to the women and families we serve. It is heartening to hear that so many women, having completed their families, have come forward to be altruistic donors after coming to know about the programme.

This is not just the start of a new programme; it is the beginning of a new chapter in the lives of countless women. And for me, it is the realisation of a vision that transcends the boundaries of traditional medicine, offering a future where the impossible becomes possible.

Mr Srjan Saso

All notable journeys begin with a serendipitous first step, and for me that was meeting the 'great Scot,' aka Professor Richard Smith, in the hallowed corridors of Hammersmith Hospital in the autumn of 2009. I was the junior doctor who had recently joined the gynaecological oncology team, and on a particularly rainy October Thursday, I was scheduled to be in theatre all day with Richard. He has always been a conversationalist, and after a day of talking about various subjects, none of them related to medicine, I found out that he was looking for a Research Fellow in a topic I had never heard about, *uterine transplantation* (UTx). At that time, I had just commenced my specialist training (or residency, as it is known in the USA) in obstetrics and gynaecology. It is rather unusual to come out of residency training to do research at such as early stage; however, Professor Smith's warmth, passion, and energy, smoothed over by his Scottish wit, did enough to point me in that direction. Of course, the topic of UTx was particularly intriguing. It was novel, science-fiction-esque, offering a philosophical challenge and combining two areas which still, to this day, excite me — surgery and fertility. I was ready to sign on the dotted line.

'Love at first sight' is not a phrase used exclusively in a romantic context. For me, this project was indeed a love story of sorts. I was enthused by the challenges of the project and wanted to work for Richard. He went on to become my PhD supervisor, with my fellowship officially beginning in 2010. It totalled three years, with most of the time spent at the Royal Veterinary College (RVC), Camden campus, and Imperial College London, South Kensington and Hammersmith Hospital campus. My other supervisor was Professor Sadaf Ghaem-Maghami. Professor Tom Bourne started me on my academic and ultrasound journey, the latter being so crucial when it comes to the science of UTx.

Multiple people helped me along the PhD journey, whether it was the physics team at the Hamlyn Centre, Imperial College London — in particular, Dr Neil Clancy and Professor Dan Elson, or the fabulous veterinary team at the RVC, Dr Michael Boyd and Professor David Noakes. There were multiple conversations, late night discussions, explanations so that I could 'get it,' a wonderfully, generous educating spirit, without any material reward. All of these people are deeply embedded in my heart, and I shall always be grateful for their support throughout. Ms Dena Kelman, Richard's personal assistant, was a constant source of laughter, joyfulness and wisdom, and I value her sincere efforts to keep me motivated with her bottomless pool of anecdotes, stories and words of advice, which helped to maintain my energy levels.

A final shout-out goes to the following: Mr Joseph Yazbek, a brother-friend, who taught me my first surgical steps and skills; Ms Maya Al-Memar, gynaecology colleague, closest confident and a pillar in my life to this day; and of course, my two oldest and best friends, Cyrus Doctor and Chris Arcoumanis, who never let me forget where I started from.

Those three years were the most exhilarating and stimulating years of my medical career. There were so many wonderful moments – but first, a quick summary of the projects.

My preliminary and first work retrospectively analysed some of the surgical work related to the *abdominal radical trachelectomy* procedure performed at our institution. This surgical procedure, invented by Professor Richard Smith, offers treatment of early-stage cervical cancer via removal of cervix with the cancer, and therefore, preservation of the body of the uterus and, in turn, the patient's fertility.

The second and third projects were animal-based and consisted of UTx in a rabbit (12-transplant) and sheep (five-transplant) model. The work focused on improving surgical technique – furthering our knowledge when it comes to the immunological response following UTx – and achieving the first ever pregnancy in a rabbit UTx model. Working with animals taught me about respect for the value of life – not just human life. Furthermore, I shall never forget the trip whereby I collected rabbit embryos from Heathrow Airport (posted by our veterinary colleagues in Valencia, Spain) to the Royal Veterinary College in Camden on the London Underground. I felt like a schoolboy – nervous, shaky, knowing that a mere slip could damage these embryos and scupper a huge amount of work, scared that I would forget them in the carriage prior to getting off. Not to mention not knowing what to say or explain in case I was accosted by the Transport Police!

The fourth study assessed methods of measuring organ viability. This work was with Professor Dan Elson and Dr Neil Clancy. The work zoned in on multispectral imaging and the application of laser-speckle contrast analysis, which is real-time, effective, and easy-to-use. Rather amusingly, the physics theory here went over my head, despite an A-level in the subject. I am therefore grateful to the physicists, especially Dr Neil Clancy, for spending many evenings with me going through the theory and helping me seem much more intelligent than I am.

The last study looked at perceptions toward UTx, both from healthcare professionals and patients. The latter group was the first time that I came across UTx patients in person. I could, therefore, truly visualise their faces, the depths of despair and the emotional turmoil that they felt. It was humbling and left a large imprint on my heart and mind. Finally, the perceptions of healthcare professionals made me understand that overall, there was support for UTx from our colleagues, further supporting our decision to persevere with this historic project.

It is also worth mentioning that, in 2012, I spent a glorious six weeks in Indianapolis, USA, under the tutelage of Professor Giuseppe Del Priore, helping to create the first ever ovarian tissue cryopreservation unit at their centre, as well as working on other avenues regarding oncofertility. This was a truly superb fellowship, and I am grateful for the opportunity. A special 'shout out' to Alexander Whitely, who I met out there and has since become a close friend, and the Slippery Noodle, the greatest bar this side of West London!

During that period, I, and the team, had to face a lot of scepticism. My response to this was that UTx was never there to replace adoption or surrogacy, but to act as a third potential option if it was deemed safe in the future. All scientists must strive to answer a question, rather than sitting on the sidelines, hypothesising, debating and philosophising. Here was our question – can UTx lead to healthy pregnancy and subsequent live birth? The answer may be 'No' in the long run, because UTx is still at the experimental stage, both with us and internationally – but at least we are trying to answer the question. The journey itself is always much more important than the end goal, and the UTx journey has resulted in plenty of clinical spin-offs and furthered our knowledge of transplant immunology, transplant surgery, fertility and gynaecology.

I was also proud to make the initial inroads and connections with NHS BT. After my PhD finished, I spent time writing it up and passed the viva in 2014, one of the proudest moments of my career and life. For that I am not only grateful to my supervisors but also my parents, my sister Anya, and my aunt without whose time, support and love, this could have never happened. They keep me on the straight and narrow, and long may it continue. I therefore dedicated my PhD to them.

As a team, we were very fortunate to have Mr Benjamin Jones join us in 2014 for the next act. He took over after me to also further research on the topic of UTx. Not only did he become a colleague, but he also then became one of my groomsmen, as well as a very close friend and confidante, and I feel very fortunate that he is in my life.

My role since 2014 has been more from a cerebral angle of offering ideas and advice. But of course, as one of the principal members of the surgical UTx team, headed by Richard, we finally completed the UK's first ever UTx in 2023, a day that will forever be etched in our collective memory bank. Twenty-four hours of tiredness, perseverance, sweat, and swearing — but for sure, composure and teamwork, to the end. Several more transplants later, we are now waiting for the first pregnancy, the principal reason for this whole journey.

A little bit about the metaphysics of this journey. The UTx journey has improved me as a person and has shown me many new sides of my character — most importantly, perseverance and not giving up, together with fortitude. I am in indebted to my family for their support and care throughout; my auntie for teaching me how to argue, my father for showing always how to keep going, whatever the obstacles; my sister for demonstrating the art of going deep when a question comes your way; and my mother for loving me, even when I did not deserve her love.

My biggest proponent was, of course, Professor Richard Smith, my mentor and second, 'work,' father. Watching this Renaissance Man work and heal has been a real privilege, and I feel truly blessed that our paths crossed in 2009.

Therefore, my last words are 'Onwards and Upwards.' We kept saying them to each other, and Richard assured me constantly that there was nothing to worry about, that we would get there eventually. I am particularly appreciative of his spirit, and most of all how he demonstrated the permanence of the following words: 'If you can trust yourself when all men doubt you/But make allowance for their doubting too.'

Onwards and Upwards, my Professor. The story of UTx has only just started in the UK and being part of the first British team to do it, helping women fulfil their fertility dreams, is something that I truly cherish and shall always honour. I am most pleased that I can now share the story of UTx with my own family – the love of my life, my wife, Karen (and her family), who puts up with my energy bursts, and my three children, who keep me grounded, and for whom all this is for: Luka, Mila and Vid.

> *Come, my friends,*
> *'Tis not too late to seek a newer world.*
> *Push off, and sitting well in order smite*
> *The sounding furrows; for my purpose holds*
> *To sail beyond the sunset, and the baths*
> *Of all the western stars, until I die.*
> *It may be that the gulfs will wash us down:*
> *It may be we shall touch the Happy Isles,*
> *And see the great Achilles, whom we knew.*
> *Tho' much is taken, much abides; and tho'*
> *We are not now that strength which in old days*
> *Moved earth and heaven, that which we are, we are;*
> *One equal temper of heroic hearts,*
> *Made weak by time and fate, but strong in will*
> *To strive, to seek, to find, and not to yield.*

Ulysses, by Alfred Lord Tennyson

Dr Saaliha Vali

Being part of the UK's first uterus transplant is an experience that transcends words – it's a journey that has redefined the boundaries of hope, science, and human resilience. It's hard to articulate the mix of emotions that come with being at the centre of such a groundbreaking procedure. There's a profound sense of gratitude, not only for the opportunity, but also for the team of dedicated medical professionals who have poured their expertise, passion, and care into making this possible.

At the same time, there's an overwhelming sense of responsibility. This isn't just a medical procedure; it's a beacon of hope for so many women who have been told that they cannot carry a child. To think that our journey could inspire or pave the way for others is both humbling and empowering. It's a reminder that, sometimes, taking on a challenge can lead to something much greater than ourselves.

As a doctor and Research Fellow on the team for over four years, the position provided me with the wonderful opportunity to be the first point of contact for the many hopeful women enquiring about their eligibility. Each case, though unique, carried a common thread of years of despair and longing for motherhood. Presenting the opportunity of a uterus transplant instilled a renewed sense of hope for women who spent years trying to accept they would never experience pregnancy. So many consultations were filled with tears as the reality of what was achievable was shared in clinic. For some this was the only route they could accept to motherhood due to personal or religious beliefs about surrogacy and adoption.

There's also a deep connection with the donors, both deceased and living — living donors whose selflessness and courage has been truly humbling, and deceased donors who have served as a reminder of the profound impact one life can have on another, especially in this context where the premature passing of one's life, such as in a tragic accident, leads to the opportunity for a couple's dream of parenthood to become a reality. Becoming a mother myself through this period has provided me with absolute clarity that this journey our patients are yearning for is worthwhile.

Yet, with all the excitement and hope, there's also the acknowledgment of the unknown. Being the first comes with uncertainties and challenges that others haven't faced. But there's also a strange comfort in that – the knowledge that I'm part of something pioneering, something that will forever change the landscape of organ transplantation and women's health.

In the end, being part of the UK's first uterus transplant feels like standing at the edge of history, where science and human spirit converge in a way that feels almost miraculous. It's an experience filled with hope, courage, and an unwavering belief in the possibilities that lie ahead.

Dr Ariadne L'Heveder

Being in the right place at the right time really pays off when you happen to walk into Mr Smith's operating theatre and his PhD student, Dr Ben Jones, is filming an experimental procedure. You start chatting about academic medicine and leave with several ideas for academic papers you're going to help their team publish. Then, six years later, you get the job as the next uterus transplant clinical Research Fellow.

When you are a very junior doctor in the UK, it is often the case that you are treated as a glorified administrative assistant. Seniors do not pay you much attention, provided that you write in the notes, order the right investigations, alert them when their patients are becoming unwell, and discharge patients in a timely manner. It is rare to be asked about your interests and future career plans.

This team, however, is different. It was February 2018, and I was a foundation year one doctor, the very first year out of medical school. I had been very lucky to secure a post as an academic foundation trainee, with protected research time in obstetrics and gynaecology at the Institute of Reproductive Developmental Biology, Imperial College London. As part of this post, I arranged a clinical week at Queen Charlotte's and Chelsea Hospital to *see* if I enjoyed the clinical aspects of obstetrics and gynaecology. On one of the days, I was meant to be on the labour ward, where women with higher-risk pregnancies would deliver their babies. One of the doctors pulled me aside and asked if I would like to go to the operating theatres instead to see an experimental surgery being performed by Mr Smith and his colleagues. I agreed; to this day, that was the best career decision I ever made.

Typically, when you are observing a surgery, particularly as a very junior doctor, you stay out of the way and keep quiet. However, shortly after walking into the operating theatre, Ben Jones started asking me questions about my role, my career and my research as part of my academic training. Knowing I needed a competitive application to secure an obstetrics and gynaecology training post in London, I was keen to try to publish some scientific papers, and Ben was full of ideas and low on time. And so began an amazing professional relationship, which continues to flourish to this day. I began writing papers on the use of ultrasound during gynaecology operations, improving IVF outcomes, obstetrics and gynaecology in elite athletes, and other topics under Ben's supervision and mentorship.

It did not take long to grasp that we worked very well together, and Ben soon started to float the idea of me joining the uterus transplant team to do my PhD. I met Mr (at the time) Smith properly for the first time, and knew he was the kind of supervisor I would love to work under – an inspiring, highly skilled and intelligent, yet completely down-to-earth person, who was also up for a laugh. Whilst I was totally flattered by the potential offer, I also had many reservations, not least the fact that I was still very early on in my career and wasn't entirely sure what I wanted to do within the field of obstetrics and gynaecology. We parked the idea, I got my training number in London and did my exams, and we continued to write papers together.

Despite Ben's protestations, as I became more experienced, I developed a keen interest in obstetrics, specifically maternal and foetal medicine, which is essentially looking after pregnant women with pre-existing or new medical conditions, and managing cases where there are concerns about the baby or babies, such as them being very small or having a problem with an organ. It was during my recent training year at University College Hospital London (UCLH), a world class maternity unit, where my career plans were really solidified. I decided I would aim to sub-specialise in maternal and foetal medicine with the aim of working in a specialist unit where I would be able to do both clinical and academic work. In order to pursue this, I would need a solid academic background and a competitive CV; naturally, the idea of doing a PhD resurfaced.

Ben and I once again raised the possibility of me joining the uterus transplant team. The current fellow's PhD was nearly finished, and a new fellow post would soon be advertised. Both the living donor and deceased donor programmes were finally up and running after a hiatus during the pandemic, and the first uterus transplant in the UK had just been performed, and the recipient and donor were both very well. This was a seriously exciting time to join the team. I knew I worked extremely well with Ben and was very excited at the opportunity to work with Professor Smith. However, the project was more focused on fertility and gynaecology than maternal-fetal medicine, and I was still slightly sceptical regarding uterus transplantation as a treatment option – did I want this to be my PhD?

As with every major career decision, I spoke to the important people around me, my now-husband, my family, friends and mentors. I give particular thanks to Tom Hirst, Carol L'Heveder, Ben Jones, Julia Turner, Julia Zöllner and Roz Augwhane for listening to me mull over the decision for hours and hours; with the latter two, these conversations were often in the middle of night, whilst delivering babies on the UCLH labour ward. On meeting Professor Smith again and discussing the project in more detail with Dr Saaliha Vali, the outgoing fellow, I knew this was an opportunity I couldn't let go. I finally made my decision; I would interview for the post and if I got the job, I would take it.

Fast-forward to August 2024, and here I am, ten months into the post and still delighted with the decision. I feel incredibly lucky to be working with such an inspiring team. Something we all share is a good sense of humour and great deal of compassion, both of which are critical when dealing with such stressful and emotional work. On meeting the transplant recipients and those seeking a uterine transplant, any degree of scepticism regarding uterus transplantation as a treatment for those with absolute uterine factor infertility has completely disappeared. This treatment changes lives and allows people to have families, something I feel is fundamental to being a human. Advancing research in women's health, an area neglected for so long, gives me some purpose, and working in this particular field is highly emotive and very exciting. I am so grateful for the doctor who took me into that operating theatre six years ago, to Ben for being so engaging and encouraging of my early academic pursuits, and finally to Professor Smith for leading such a fantastic team.

Miss Ann Ogbemudia

Very early in my general surgery training, I knew that transplant surgery was the specialty for me. There is something special, unique, and almost sacred about transplant surgery.

In deceased-donor donation, accepted donations are mostly from healthy donors, meaning their death is usually unexpected — a traumatizing experience for those involved. In their darkest moment, the loved ones of the deceased dig deep to help others, despite their fresh grief. This is the highest form of altruism, sharing a part of their loved one to help unknown strangers, with identities protected on both sides.

The situation of the organ recipients is also unique. They accept this gift from a stranger — a bittersweet gift. Amid their hope to become better and have a second chance at life, they are acutely aware of the cost of this gift. There is no other surgical specialty filled with such love, pain, hope, innovation, and ethical conundrums.

I clearly remember being approached by our Chair and Professor of Transplantation, Professor Peter Friend. He is a man who remarkably hides his sparkling intelligence under a cloak of humility. We had a meeting in his office to discuss potential topics for my PhD. Looking at me intently, with his fingers pressed together, he said, 'How about uterus perfusion?' I stared back, gave a small smile, and replied that I would do some preliminary research into its potential. However, what I really thought was, 'Whatever for?!'

Under Professor Friend's guidance, our Oxford unit had gained world-class recognition for innovation – among other things, for the development of liver perfusion, which irrevocably transformed liver preservation for transplantation. Similarly, kidney perfusion was being developed to increase organ availability and improve transplant outcomes. 'Speak to Isabel Quiroga-Giraldez,' Professor Friend said, with a twinkle in his eye. Our meeting ended, and speak to Miss Quiroga-Giraldez I did.

Isabel cut no corners. 'Our goal with uterus transplantation is to provide women a chance to carry life themselves. We can do this. It's time,' she said. I raised my eyebrows – I admit I was sceptical. I needed a moment to grasp the need for this type of transplantation. I was used to transplants for life-saving health conditions: kidney failure, diabetes, liver failure – the need for heart and lungs in order to live.

Additionally, I admit, I am not a mother, and many of my female friends in surgery do not have children. It's an unspoken truth that we all know – an inadvertent sacrifice made for our surgical careers. Not having yet experienced the intrinsic yearning for motherhood, my empathy switch wasn't fully on. But my scientific switch was, so I smiled back and gave an enthusiastic cheer: 'Let's do it!' Little did I know I was about to embark on a transformative journey myself.

I met with the gynaecology group – our other half! – Professor Richard Smith, Dr Ben Jones, and Dr Saaliha Vali. Richard was philosophical and jovial, Ben was ambitious and Rabelaisian, and Saaliha was the heart of the team. We were a good match, a good blend of characters for making this happen.

For many years, they had worked relentlessly with animal models, joined other uterus transplant groups, sought ethics approvals, and raised funds, undergoing massive efforts to ensure the first uterus transplant in the UK happened.

Then, COVID-19 took the world, and the transplant community, by surprise. Patients awaiting transplants, with their hope for health, were put on hold, and difficult decisions had to be made in prioritising access to hospital care alongside the critical COVID-19 patients. It was a difficult time. The uterus transplant programme came to a halt — a blow to all the hard work that had finally gained momentum.

Eventually, the tide turned, and the world began to recover. We returned to our usual practice. I had almost forgotten, until I received a text from Isabel one evening: 'Are you ready for the first living donor uterus transplant?' 'It's happening,' I thought. 'YES.'

On that day, I met the families of the donor and recipient. It was a necessity for me — not just as a surgeon (you always meet your patients multiple times prior to surgery), but as a person. Meeting them humanised why we were doing this, and what we were doing this for.

I met the sisters; the older sister was donating to her younger sister. I thought about my younger brother, who similarly is a few years younger than me. Despite the usual sibling squabbles, I knew he adored me, looked up to me, and tried to emulate me.

I imagined them as children, with the younger one, one day noticing that she was not having the same experiences as her older sister. When would her menstrual period arrive? I imagined her eventually receiving the news from the doctor that she was different from her older sister, different from her mother, and different from womankind. She was different. She deserved this — the full journey of motherhood. Her sister wanted this for her too, and was ready to undergo surgical risk for her. I was committed, heart and soul, to the task at hand.

That shift in my mindset was necessary, because the surgeries were long, emotional rollercoasters, and a real test of our physical endurance. We started in the morning and finished the next morning. We were committed and locked in — for her, for others like her, and for the undoubtedly loved children this procedure would bring.

Sister Lian Lee

The following note and poems were written to Isabel shortly after the momentous events that Sister Lee, Deputy Matron, so much contributed to: the living donor transplant. The team would like to share them here in acknowledgement of her dedication and care.

> Dear Isabel,
>
> It is an honour and humbling experience to be among the amazing teams and talented individuals! Hope you find meaning in the poem, which is a true reflection of my pride and gratitude to everyone as a nurse and a nurse leader.
>
> Poetry is a way of my expressing the life experiences, and to capture those beautiful moments.
>
> Thanks again for the opportunity to be in the journey.
>
> With best regards,
> Lian

The Transformation of Life

The long-awaited Sunday morning finally arrived
Sisters, husband, and parents meet the surgeons
A day of hope, every parent's wish
Humanity meets ground-breaking surgery

A group of compassionate professionals
Energised and high-spirited with only one goal
A moment shared with ambitions and imagination
Organ transplantation, hope for many

Gentle surgeons with delicate hands
Scalpel, tools, and sutures to mention a few
Eyes fixed on every blood vessel and organ
Only the 'loupe' can reveal hope beneath

Silence tells the story in the operating room
Eyes and ears focussed on the screens
Every alarm from the machine alerts, life under the drape
Second minutes count as time passes by

136

An elegant display of every surgical movement
Intelligence meets technologies; marriage of art and science
The melodious soft music in the background
Calms the souls in an intense life-saving space

The operating room transforms into a magical theatre
It brings life in the sterile space, a monumental experience
The spirit of pride and grace lingers in the air
The story shall continue only few realise as they journey onwards

Later, in July 2023, Sister Lee reflected on the surgery, and the impact that it had on her.

Hi Isabel,

I have the privilege to reflect on the journey and experience shared that you and the Imperial team and our amazing Churchill theatre's team had embarked upon. As you all have celebrated the hope that the experts have given to the lady and family. I like to honour the moment, as I recorded in this poem, to pay my deepest gratitude to the dedication from all of you. Life and hope from sterile space transformed with magical movement to lift the soul!!

I hope you and colleagues find meanings in this humble poem recording the rhythm that everyone has created.

Lian

Rhythm of Life

There is a soul in every heart
Encouragement, hope and grace
Constant companion despite obstacles
Shower of blessing and gratitude, they pray

Wisdom of courage, only they realise
Darkness and uncertainty they concur
The light within shines the brightest
Reward to the souls once crossed the line

The power of imagination lifts the souls
Lightness they feel, life and hope give
Vulnerability they embrace
The spirit of life, they breathe

Magical transformation, they co-create
Melodious lyrics, elegantly staged
Beautiful moments they shared in the sterile space
Graciously the souls dance the rhythm of life

About a year later, Sister Lee shared one further poem following the lecture entitled 'The first human womb transplant in the UK' that Richard and Isabel gave at the Royal Institution in June 2024 (see Chapter 3).

An Epic Journey

Storms, they brave.
Courage, they strive.
Conversation sparks
Debates linger.

Two aspiring professionals
Physician and surgeon
Future generations, they inspire
Illuminating lecture

The Ri, a prestigious theatre
Wooden arc desk, motivational speeches
life, hope and mission.
The birth of innovations

Silence fills the room.
A magical moment
Heartbeats intensify.
Eager souls await.

Stories shared in the room.
Audiences intently listen.
Eyes they look on.
Beautiful minds, passionate individuals.

Smartly, they dress.
The warmth they radiate.
Innovation, they co-produce
The sprout of hope, their compassion

Majestic stage, science meets humanity.
An epic journey, accompanied by many.
Diligently and professionally
Tears of joy, kind seeds they sow.

The souls and family look back.
A priceless gift, a seed of kindness
Rain nurture as the sky opens.
Rainbows remind, hope after the storm.

• Part IV •
Future Research and Considerations

Chapter

11

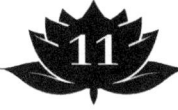

Legal and
Ethical Considerations

Ethical Considerations Relating to Uterine Transplantation

In the late 1990s, there was much discussion regarding the ethics of performing uterine transplantation. We were blessed with three advisors, the late Dr Andrew Lawson, Mr Martin Lupton, and Professor Raanan Ghillon, all of Imperial College. They broke things down, utilising the four pillars of medical ethics:

1. *Primum non nocere*: first, do no harm. This is also called non-maleficence, or the duty to 'not do bad.'
2. Beneficence: the duty to do good.
3. Autonomy: respect for the patient's right to self-determination.
4. Justice: to treat all people equally and equitably.

When one thinks about uterine transplantation in these terms, we may fall down with respect to the first pillar. We are proposing IVF, followed, if successful, by major surgery to implant the uterus, one or two Caesarean sections, and then a completion hysterectomy. All this incorporates immunosuppression over a two-to-five-year period. Admittedly, however, we are not alone in walking the line on these pillars; in pursuit of 2, 3 and 4, much of modern medicine, particularly surgery, chemotherapy, and radiotherapy fall short. We start to score much more highly with the second pillar — beneficence. We are, with uterine transplantation, seeking the begetting of children, which is a key element in human flourishing, itself a central goal of all medicine.

Autonomy encompasses respect for the sentient patient's wishes, in particular having confirmed that the putative patient understands the risks and benefits of the proposed procedure(s). In respect to our research, we have met hundreds of well-balanced women who desire this operation and who understand, and are well informed of, the risks involved. For the record, these are risks of infection, deep venous thrombosis (DVT), haemorrhage, anaesthesia, and other organ damage. These risks apply to each of the proposed operations that each woman will need to go through. Specific to the uterine transplant itself is the risk of graft failure, rejection, and the risks associated with immuno-suppressive therapy — namely, of cancer and infection. Admittedly, as in any new technique, there are the unknown risks, something that the patient needs to be aware of. This is now much less of an issue for the living-donor transplant method, as enough have been performed that we are aware of most risks, but it is still an issue for deceased-donor transplant, hence its trial status.

Having said all of this, we take specific steps to reduce each risk: prophylactic (preventative) antibiotics for infection; blood thinners to reduce the risk of DVT; and appropriate surgical technique to reduce the risk of haemorrhage and other organ damage. Good-quality anaes-thesia is a given for our patients, and the graft will be in for less than five years. Unlike with a vital organ transplant, such as the liver, a uterus graft will be in the patient's body relatively temporarily, and if the graft fails it is not life-threatening, because it is not a vital organ. The non-vital nature of the uterus allows for its removal to reduce risks for the patient if those circumstances occur. Additionally, those patients undergoing vital organ transplant are by their very nature unwell people, hence their need for transplant; the opposite is true of our patients, who are debarred from the uterine transplant programme if they have intercurrent medical conditions.

The final pillar of medical ethics is justice, a concept familiar to all of us. As with the second pillar, justice is a driver towards helping women without a uterus achieve pregnancy and motherhood.

Legal and Regulatory Aspects of Uterus Transplantation in the UK

While surrogacy offers the possibility of having biological children, it remains prohibited or heavily restricted in many countries due to ethical, religious, or legal concerns. In the UK, surrogacy is legal, yet commercial surrogacy is banned, leading to a shortage of available surrogates. Moreover, the legal landscape surrounding surrogacy is uncertain, as the law designates the woman who carries and gives birth to the child as the legal mother. Additionally, surrogacy agreements lack legal binding and are unenforceable if the surrogate changes her mind after birth, creating enormous uncertainty and anxiety amongst intended parents. Adoption provides an alternative pathway to parenthood, albeit without biological relatedness. However, it presents its own set of challenges, including rigorous assessments and vetting of prospective parents, lengthy waiting periods, and no guarantee of being matched with a child.

Uterine transplantation stands as the sole option capable of anatomically and physiologically restoring fertility in women with uterine factor infertility, offering the potential for biological, legal, and social parenthood. This procedure merges elements of assisted reproduction technology and organ transplantation, navigating regulatory frameworks set forth by statutes like the Human Fertilisation and Embryology (HFE) Act of 1990, the Human Tissue Act of 2004, and the Human Organ (Deemed Consent) Act of 2019. In England, regulating uterine transplantation akin to other organ transplants would align it with the Human Tissue Act of 2004 and the Human Organ Act of 2019, depending on whether the uterus is sourced from a living or deceased donor. The Human Tissue Authority (HTA) serves as the statutory body overseeing the removal, storage, use, and disposal of human bodies, organs, and tissues for various purposes, including transplantation.

The National Health Service organ donor register boasts 25 million registered individuals. In May 2020, a significant change to organ donation law in England for deceased donation occurred with the implementation of the Organ Donation (Deemed Consent) Act (2019), ushering in an 'opt-out' system. Under this framework, adults are automatically presumed to consent to organ or tissue donation when they die, unless they have explicitly chosen to opt out. However, like other rare or novel transplant procedures such as limb and face transplants, the donation of the uterus is not covered by the opt-out strategy. As such, explicit consent from the family, close friend, or nominated representative of the deceased donor is required. Yet, obtaining proxy consent during an emotionally tumultuous period presents significant challenges, with grieving families often hesitant to proceed with donation if the deceased individual's wishes regarding organ donation were not known.

The Human Tissue Act of 2004 mandates that all transplants involving living donors must receive approval from the Human Tissue Authority. Prior to surgery, the living donor undergoes meticulous preoperative interviews, including psychological assessments, to confirm that she has completed her family and fully comprehends the implications of donating her uterus, including the potential loss of future gestational capability. Once the medical team confirms the donor's suitability, an independent assessor steps in to verify compliance with the Human Tissue Act of 2004, safeguarding the donor's interests and ensuring that no coercion or incentive has influenced the decision.

Living donation can be directed (when the donor knows the recipient), or non-directed (when the recipient is unknown to the donor). The same principles apply to both directed and non-directed living donors – provided there is explicit consent, absence of coercion, and no financial compensation involved, altruistic donation is permissible.

While there are no specific age restrictions for living donors, concerns may arise regarding young women, particularly those without prior childbirth experience, who wish to donate their uterus. These concerns underscore the need for careful consideration and ethical evaluation in such cases.

Whilst at the time of writing, we are only considering directed donation for our living donor cases, we are looking to open up the donation process to non-directed donors in the near future. For every email received from the charity from a woman seeking a uterus transplant, we receive emails from three women offering to donate their uterus to help others. It has been highly frustrating not being able to accept these generous offers, but we are hopeful that we will soon be able to.

In light of the number of women approaching the charity, we undertook a study to explore their motivations and perceptions in donating their uterus for transplantation. 152 women responded. Their primary motivations included the desire to help others experience childbirth and a sense of altruism. Despite recognising the risks involved, many respondents remained enthusiastic about donation. However, when we applied our selection criteria, fewer than a third of them were suitable to proceed with the procedure, highlighting the need for careful consideration in donor selection. Overall, we found that women who consider uterine donation anticipate psychological and emotional benefits from enabling another woman to conceive and give birth, despite the physical risks of the donation procedure and its potential impact on their daily activities.

The legal status of a transplanted uterus is another subject requiring consideration, particularly in cases involving live donors. The possibility of a live donor changing her mind and requesting the uterus back, even after it has served its intended purpose, raises legal questions surrounding organ restitution. Some legal scholars argue that human tissue, once detached from the body, becomes a tangible entity subject to property rights. Under this view, the uterus would be considered the property of the donor until it is implanted into the recipient, at which point ownership would transfer to the recipient. However, given its temporary therapeutic function, others question whether the uterus should be treated more like an implantable medical device, where ownership after removal remains with the surgical team. English law currently lacks specific regulations addressing organ restitution, likely because most organ transplants have historically been permanent.

While the Human Tissue Authority provides guidance on the living donor's right to withdraw consent before transplantation, it does not address withdrawal of consent post-transplantation. Donors are typically given options regarding the disposition of the organ if it is not implanted into the intended recipient. Once transplanted, the uterus, like any other organ, requires explicit consent from the recipient before removal. In cases of organ restitution, the original recipient would be treated as a donor under the law, subject to the same organ donation policies.

Finally, the legal considerations surrounding children born from a donor uterus also warrant careful examination. Currently, the Human Fertilisation and Embryology Authority does not provide specific guidelines regarding the legal status of uterus donors. However, under existing laws, once the recipient successfully conceives and gives birth following uterine transplantation, the child legally belongs to her, similar to the legal framework governing surrogacy. This aspect of uterus transplantation alleviates some of the legal complexities associated with surrogacy and adoption, as the donor relinquishes any legal rights over the resulting child.

While the offspring of uterus transplant recipients will share genetic traits with their recipient parents, who of course provided the gametes, questions remain regarding the potential presence of the uterus donor's DNA in subsequent offspring. Limited research exists on this topic, although there are suggestions that the lining of the uterus, the endometrium, may influence the genetic makeup of the embryo. Evidence indicates that molecules present in the endometrial fluid can impact the embryo's development by modifying it. This concept raises important scientific considerations regarding the potential transmission of genetic material from the donor to the offspring, necessitating further research to clarify distinctions between recipient parents and donors.

Chapter

12

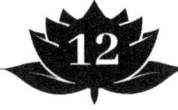

A Look to the Future

Whole Body Image and Transgender Women

We have left this aspect to the end of the book, since it encompasses some of the rationale for both women assigned female at birth and transgender women. The purpose of our programme has always been to allow women without a uterus the opportunity to carry their own baby. And, as one talks to the women, one of the things that often comes up is that they don't feel whole without a womb — something that was also demonstrated in our survey amongst transgender women. Of course, we are only foreseeing the new uterus being implanted for a maximum of five years to ensure maximum safety. There is a clear tension and dichotomy in this, which I think is unanswerable until organ transplantation comes without the need for immunosuppression.

From an ethical standpoint, the consideration of uterine transplantation in transgender women is driven by principles of justice and equality. Just like in women assigned female at birth, transgender women may experience psychological distress due to a misalignment between their reproductive capacity and aspirations. The inability to undergo gestation, a fundamental aspect of female identity for many, can be deeply impactful and transformative, and may continue to negatively impact the mental health of transgender women following transition.

Legally, transgender individuals are protected from discrimination under the Equality Act (2010), which explicitly prohibits both direct and indirect forms of discrimination based on gender reassignment alone. This means that transgender women cannot be discriminated against solely because of their gender identity.

As uterine transplantation becomes a recognised treatment option for women assigned female at birth, UK legislation would make it legally unacceptable to deny the procedure to transgender women on the basis of their gender identity without sufficient reason. This underscores the importance of ensuring equitable access to reproductive healthcare for all individuals, regardless of gender identity.

That said, performing uterus transplant in this population raises a number of anatomical, physiological, fertility and obstetric considerations that would undoubtedly necessitate significant further research into the concept. There is no doubting in our minds that the media has raised false expectations for transgender women in this respect. This whole book, which has described our 25 years of effort, is effectively showing that we adhered to a concept called Moore's Criteria for surgical innovation. This involves determining whether there is a population of people likely to benefit that have any desire to undergo the procedure; then to basic animal research; then to gauging professional and public attitudes; then human cadaveric work; only then is the procedure introduced to patients in a well-ordered and ethically acceptable trial. This we have done for women born as women; there is virtually no work in this area that has been performed in the transgender setting, and we would agree with Mats Brännström's recent publication, which placed this development 10–20 years away.

Thus, prior to commencing any animal-based work, we felt it was essential to gauge demand amongst transgender women to determine whether or not there was a need to pursue this area.

In 2019, Ben and I finished in the operating theatre and after some administrative work got into the car to go to the South Kensington campus of Imperial College London. Ben had submitted an ethics application to the Imperial College London Research Ethics Committee to undertake a survey study gauging the reproductive aspirations of transgender women and their perceptions of uterine transplantation. As we drove, he said, 'Mr Smith, have you read this Ethics Proposal?' To which I replied 'Er, no, I think you had better fill me in.'

We duly arrived at the college and parked up. As we got in the lift, I wrote three things on my hand – 1995, 2016 and 2010. There was quite a queue of anxious researchers outside the meeting room – including us. A few minutes later, we were called and entered a very small room with a relatively large number of people in it. There were two empty seats which we sat down in. Most of the committee were casually dressed, but I was in a suit and coat, and Ben was in a smart jacket. The Chairman introduced himself as the Professor of a Mathematical subject, and then asked who we were. I replied 'I'm Richard Smith and this is Ben Jones. I'm a gynaecological surgeon and he's my PhD fellow.' The Chairman then said, 'We'd better tell you who we are.' Round the table we went. First came another Mathematics professor, then a professor of Retrovirology, then the Curator of the Natural History Museum, then the head of all medical research at Imperial College London, a student representative and so on. Quite staggering that all these luminaries should be in this tiny, sweaty room, and even more amazing they should be considering our very modest little questionnaire.

The Chairman then said, 'We are in a hurry this evening, running late, and you will need to be quick – you have three minutes to tell us your project.' Now normally, Ben does more of the talking at these things than I do, but this time round, that would not have been fair – this place felt like a bear pit. So, I replied: 'In 1995, I started research into uterine transplant. I'm a gynaecological cancer surgeon, so we always saw this as a treatment for women with no uterus. Then in 2016, we went to a full two-day conference on the ethics of uterine transplant. At this conference, we discovered the 2010 Gender Equality Act, which mandates equal care for transgender women as for cisgender women.

So, before we embark on a series of animal-based research projects, we would like to know if the transgender community are interested in this possibility, hence our survey.' Our presentation was over in less than a minute.

The look on the committee's faces was a picture. The Chairman said, 'any questions?' There were none. And he then said, 'That's it, you are out of here, we will let you know tomorrow.' Feeling like we were speed dating, Ben and I left, nodded to the rest of the queue, and did a high five, before heading to the nearest bar for a gin and tonic. The following day we got the go-ahead — and what interesting results we obtained.

In this study, we gave transgender women an online questionnaire to better understand their reproductive aspirations and plans, and gauge their perceptions and motivations regarding uterus transplant. Around 180 transgender women responded, each contributing a unique voice to the discourse on gender identity and reproductive choices. The cohort were primarily in their twenties, with the majority expressing a longing for parenthood and only a small minority having had children prior to their transition. Their yearning for future offspring echoed through the data, emphasizing a deeply rooted desire for familial connection and biological continuity. This group of trans-gender women in particular shared a profound desire to embrace physiological experiences often reserved for women assigned female at birth. Gestation, childbirth, and menstruation emerged as symbols of femininity, with over 90% of respondents believing that such experi-ences would enhance their sense of womanhood. Our study also highlighted a complex interplay between physical and psychological well-being. Participants envisioned undergoing uterus transplant not only as a means of fulfilling their reproductive dreams, but also as a pathway to improved quality of life and happiness. Despite the sobering reality of the inherent risks involved and uncertainties that accom-pany such a major and novel procedure, many transgender women viewed the potential benefits as outweighing them. Given the novelty and significance of our findings, they were published in *JAMA Network Open*. The full manuscript can be found open access online.

Having utilised the paper that came from our survey, the question had been answered as to the wishes of the transgender female community in no uncertain terms. This led to much discussion within the group as to feasibility on many different levels. From an anatomical perspective, the unique pelvic anatomy of transgender women post-gender reassignment surgery introduces complexities that require meticulous consideration to ensure compatibility and functionality post-transplantation.

When considering the pelvic bones, it is worthwhile considering that differences between male and female pelvises are significant enough that they can be used to determine gender during autopsy. This variation has evolved due to specific selection pressures related to each sex's unique physiological needs. For instance, males require a pelvis suited for bipedal locomotion, while females need one spacious enough to accommodate a growing foetus during pregnancy and facilitate childbirth. While skeletal measurements tend to be larger in males overall, the female pelvis has evolved to be larger and broader. Moreover, in females, the pelvic inlet is oval-shaped, whereas in males, it is heart-shaped. These anatomical differences may predispose female transgender individuals post-uterine transplant to an issue whereby the foetal head is too big to descend through the pelvis, if they were to attempt labour. However, given the concerns about the mechanical strain of labour, Caesarean section is the recommended mode of delivery for women post-uterine transplant, and the same would apply to transgender women.

This brings us onto the potential issues that may arise due to issues related to the microbiome of the vagina. In the vast majority of cases of uterine transplantation undertaken so far, the recipient's vagina has been surgically connected to a vaginal cuff, which varies in length and is obtained as part of the graft. This procedure not only restores reproductive anatomy but also enables the natural excretion of fluids and menstrual flow. Importantly, it allows direct visualisation of the cervix and facilitates the taking of biopsies, which is crucial for detecting rejection following the procedure. All transgender women who have a vagina have a neovagina. In the transgender setting, a neovagina, or 'new vagina,' is created following removal of the testicles and penis, and the creation of a clitoris, labia and vagina, usually with tissue from the penis. While the inverted penile tissue is the standard method for constructing a neovagina, alternatives include using intestinal or pelvic peritoneal tissue, particularly in cases of penoscrotal hypoplasia, which can be induced by feminizing hormones. However, the small number of transplanted patients who had a neovagina, i.e., an artificially constructed vagina, have fared badly, with multiple miscarriages – so much so that a neovagina is an absolute preclusion for our programme for women born as women.

However, in either case, the absence of a physiologically functional vaginal mucosa undoubtedly poses significant challenges. The lining of the vagina serves as a barrier against microorganisms and plays a role in recognising and eliminating pathogens, contributing to the establishment of a healthy microbial flora dominated by lactobacilli, which helps prevent infections and maintain pregnancy. In transgender women, penile skin-lined neovaginas have elevated pH levels due to the inability to support the growth of acidic lactobacilli, leading to colonisation by bacteria from skin or intestinal microflora. Consequently, following uterus transplant in transgender women, the presence of a skin or intestinal neovagina, combined with immunosuppression, may increase susceptibility to recurrent vaginal infections and create an environment unsuitable for sustaining pregnancy, leading to a high miscarriage rate.

To address this anatomical challenge, a utero-vaginal transplant could be considered in this setting, using as much donor vagina as possible, along with the uterus. This would involve a technique similar to that used in radical hysterectomy, but given the increased radicality, this approach would necessitate retrieval from deceased donors. Alternatively, transgender men undergoing hysterectomy and vaginectomy could potentially serve as donors, although the increased complexity of the procedure may pose challenges and ethically unacceptable risks to the donor.

Interestingly, with regard to the prospect of having a transplanted vagina, our questionnaire study demonstrated that more than 90% felt that a functioning transplanted vagina would improve their sex life, quality of life and help them to feel like 'more of a woman.'

With regards to the blood vessels, the feasibility of retrieving a graft from a female donor and implanting it into a transgender female recipient's pelvis necessitates a detailed understanding of the intersex differences in pelvic vascular anatomy. Studies have shown that while there may be no significant difference in the length of internal iliac arteries between sexes, there is a discrepancy in vessel calibre, with female vessels being slightly wider than male vessels. These are the blood vessels removed with the graft. This disparity could potentially predispose to thrombosis, but careful surgical techniques, such as anastomosing at proximal points where vessel sizes are more similar, should help mitigate this risk. Additionally, data from lower-limb angioplasties (a procedure used to widen narrowed or obstructed blood vessels) suggest that there is no significant difference between sexes in calibre of the external iliac artery (the vessels used to connect the uterus during the implantation), further informing the surgical approach for uterine transplantation in transgender women.

In the journey of transition, discussions about fertility preserva-tion should take precedence before embarking on hormone therapy or considering gender reassignment surgery. For those seeking to preserve their fertility before transitioning, sperm cryopreservation offers a pathway to have biologically related children. Later, *in vitro* fertilization (IVF) can be undertaken, using either a female partner if they have one, or donor eggs. After uterus transplant, pregnancy may become attain-able using the same hormone regimens that have been proven effective in women with premature ovarian insufficiency or postmenopausal conditions to ensure the inside lining of the transplanted uterus is receptive to the embryo.

In conclusion, the decision to pursue uterine transplantation as part of gender reassignment surgery in transgender individuals requires careful consideration of anatomical, hormonal, fertility, and obstetric factors. However, prior to embarking on uterus transplant in transgender women, much further research is imperative if we are to come anywhere close to fulfilling Moore's criteria described above. This includes cadaveric retrieval and implantation studies to assess anatomical feasibility, as well as revisiting animal studies to uncover potential unknown risks and determine the viability of conception and pregnancy maintenance in genetic males.

Whilst the possibility of performing uterine transplantation in transgender women raises certain legal issues, there are also other key legal and regulatory implications for performing uterine transplantation in the UK. To our minds, the media have raised false hopes within the transgender community in a scientifically inaccurate fashion. To conclude, if it is to be performed responsibly, Moore's criteria for surgical innovation need to be fulfilled, and that is many years away.

Extracorporeal Gestation

This has been a concept for decades; babies grown in machines! This is where one may be tipping into Frankensteinian science. However, before we leap to that conclusion, consider that there are women with cardiac anomalies who are told that if they fall pregnant, they have a 50% chance of death. Many of these women still go ahead and become pregnant, and sadly 50% of them do die in pursuit of motherhood. Whilst surrogacy provides an option, the limitations associated with it, such as the legal and religious implications and shortage of surrogates, make it unsuitable or unacceptable to many. Might not these women be helped if their babies could be grown in a machine?

We made a very early connection with Organox, a company that produces normothermic perfusion devices that are used in organ transplantation. Whereas organs are traditionally kept cold, or on ice, to prevent damage to cells, these devices perfuse the organ at body temperature, which is a more logical approach if tissue damage can be prevented. It offers a number of advantages, most notably the avoidance or minimisation of cold ischaemic injury, but also offers the ability to monitor the condition of the organ whilst it is being perfused, to ensure it is suitable to be used. Better still, it permits the perfusion of additives and therapies to facilitate resuscitation and optimisation of the organ prior to transplantation. Finally, organ transplantation from deceased donors is an urgent operation, with obvious logistical challenges, but the ability to preserve organs for longer periods allows semi-elective planning, which could help streamline clinical care. Normothermic perfusion technology has been successfully used in transplantation of livers, kidneys, hearts and lungs.

We got involved with Organox to see if it could offer similar advantages in uterus transplant – namely, to enhance the quality of the uterus, and time the implantation more favourably around NHS operating lists, the teams' busy schedules.

When we were undertaking our rabbit model studies, we determined that the gestation period of a rabbit was around a month. As our brains can't help but think outside the box, we hypothesised that if we could keep a uterus viable for that time, it may be possible to maintain a pregnancy *ex vivo*. On one of our trips to Valencia, we undertook a series of experiments to assess if it was possible to perfuse a rabbit uterus. Our first study was successful, but there was an area between 10 and 12 o'clock where the graft was not being perfused optimally.

The study was repeated in another graft, and an excellent circuit was created, demonstrating that it is indeed possible to perfuse a rabbit uterus. Blue dye was used to check the flow through the vessels.

Whilst this concept is in its infancy and requires significant further work, we intend to undertake a further study perfusing the graft with blood, using advanced temperature control, and the addition of an oxygenator to the circuit, to determine how long a rabbit uterus can remain viable.

Further Possibilities

The golden rule with trying to look into the future is you are likely to be wrong. The history of medicine is riven with startling advances that can almost sweep away entire specialities; sometimes new things arise that turn things on their head. Two recent examples are antibiotics arriving on the scene in the 1940s and infectious diseases (ID) seemingly disappearing as a result. Glasgow had 2,000 hospital beds in the 1970s devoted to ID that were decommissioned; then by the 90s HIV had arrived necessitating many more ID beds; and then just look at COVID-19. None of these things were foreseen. The other example is interventional cardiologists, physicians 'stealing the pants off' the cardiac surgeons, with many of the latter being forced to re-train. Authors beware, because whatever you write may be held up to ridicule in future! However, it is impossible not to make a few guesses.

Extracorporeal pregnancy, as discussed above, has some prospects, but of course so much of what this book has been about is in fact satisfying women's desires to gestate. We have written much on both cisgender and transgender women. Treatment has become a real possibility for an ever-increasing number of cisgender women. As we have discussed, there is likely to be a shortage of deceased donors to meet the demand, and in time we believe that the addition of an altruistic living-donation programme will ensure sustainability in the future.

Currently, performing uterine transplant in transgender women is inappropriate until much further research confirms its feasibility. However, looking forward a good few years, one can see that the current issues are likely to be overcome, making it possible.

Tissue engineering clearly holds the key to much success in future. The creation of bioengineered uteruses appears to be many years away, but does not seem impossible. Maxine's project (Chapter 6) sets the scene in the future for the prevention of Asherman's syndrome and all the misery it causes. Absolute uterine factor infertility related to hysterectomy as treatment for cancer is likely to become far less common as the new immunotherapies evolve across the cancer field, resulting in far fewer surgeries overall, including hysterectomies.

As a team, we have also conceived of the idea of preserving the Fallopian tubes or utilizing the Fallopian tubes of the recipient to avoid the need for IVF, which is a huge cost consideration in the overall project. Women with MRKH, though lacking a uterus, usually have pristine Fallopian tubes. The fact they do not have a uterus has ironically protected their tubes from any ascending infection, and the lack of uterus has protected them from endometriosis – these two factors being the commonest causes of tubal infertility. Using a recipient's Fallopian tubes does, however, increase the risk of ectopic pregnancy.

Another possible area is that of tissue freezing. This is where tissue is frozen, allowing storage long term. This is a reality with small pieces of tissue like human eggs and embryos. If uteruses could be frozen, it would allow for their long-term storage, and a bank could then be built of uteruses for implantation at a date convenient to the recipient and the surgical team. This, of course, would be a revolution across the whole of transplant surgery.

For the UK's own programmes, with all the resources of NHSBT, we have fallen way behind the rest of the world in living-donor transplant. However, in the field of deceased-donor uterine transplant, we do have the capacity, in the future, for one of the biggest programmes in the world.

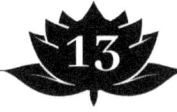

13

Conclusions

Womb Transplant UK's story has been an amazing thing to be part of. We always seek to collaborate with anybody who approaches us with good ideas. This has led to a remarkable number of fascinating projects, with many trainees obtaining postgraduate degrees helping them on their career pathway or leading them to stay within the team — the cause of science having been advanced by increments. COVID-19 casts a long shadow, not least in the way medical scientists now often interact virtually rather than face-to-face.

There is no doubting this makes great sense in the clinical field — for example, in multidisciplinary team (MDT) meetings, Zoom and Microsoft Teams allow the Oxford and Imperial Teams to meet efficiently to discuss patient management without the travel between the two cities that would otherwise be required. This has the advantage of saving both time and carbon footprint. The same argument is utilised when it comes to medical conferences.

As we hope this book has shown, there is, however, nothing that has quite beat face-to-face contact. Most of the collaborations described in this book came about directly from meeting people and subsequently dining with them at conferences. Relationships form, deals are struck, and good work progresses. In addition, fun is had in the process. This is not a trendy thing to write, but it is vitally important to keeping a team going over the years of advances and failures that form the normal vicissitudes of scientific progress. We hope that the multitude of personal anecdotes in the book have brought out the fun that has been had in search of the goals. No group could sustain this length of process without having at least a little fun and some successes.

Much of this conviviality, for our team, has revolved around food. Communal eating used to be encouraged in hospitals in the UK. Up until 30 years ago most medical teams ate together regularly at lunch time. This is still the case in Europe. If a team eat together, whether it's a picnic in the operating department or sitting down to dine, it always brings them together, encouraging free, non-hierarchal discourse. For every surgery involved in the womb transplant process, the team has shared a picnic. In the shot below, we catch a glimpse of the large quantities of food consumed, as well as the many smiling faces — all knowing they are likely to be in the operating theatre for an insane amount of time!

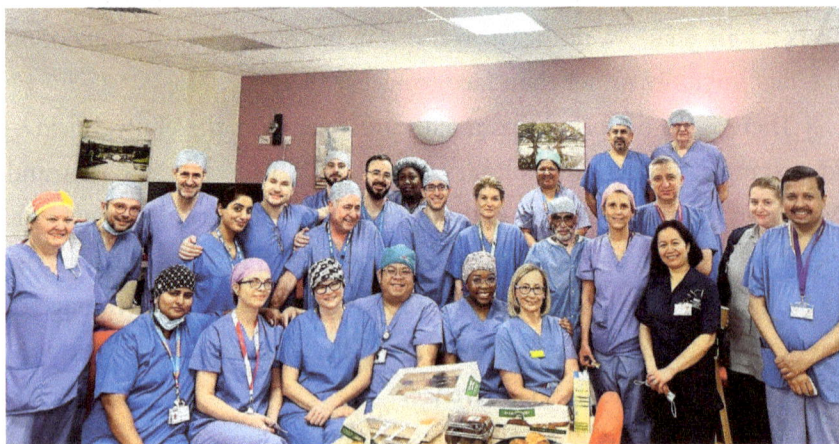

A team picnic!

One of the amazing things about the team that we never fully realised until we started operating together is their confluence of surgical skills. The cancer surgeon aims to remove a diseased organ with a 1 cm margin of normal tissue surrounding it and then to send it to histopathology for analysis. This involves the sealing/occluding the organ's blood supply, which can utilise a variety of techniques. The transplant surgeon removes a healthy organ, with no margin of normal tissue, but with as many pristine blood vessels as possible, to insert into another patient. This juxtaposition of skills is essential in uterine transplantation, surgery without ego between the teams being an essential element. The team are all co-dependent on each other for a successful outcome.

We believe that our continued focus on absolute uterine factor infertility is a great strength that has prevented dilution of our effort and helped to arrive at a place of some success. We have discovered, with only four patients currently transplanted, that this involves a huge ongoing effort across the team utilising a multitude of skills. The MDT includes transplant surgeons, pharmacology and virology, and within gynaecology, IVF, early pregnancy, immunology, high risk obstetrics, nephrology, immunology – not to mention histopathology and radiology. We all feel it's a great privilege to be part of this great endeavour.

We are very fortunate as team to be supported by the charity, Womb Transplant UK, and we express our gratitude to our patrons, the Baroness Cox, Mr Nick Maughan CBE and Ms Nadine Kaneva, and also to the myriad of people who have run charity events, marathons and the like in our support. It is that support that allows and encourages us not let go of the multiplicity of good ideas and novel developments that keep appearing.

Our team motto has always been 'Collaboration, collaboration, collaboration.' This has served us well. As Isabel said in her Royal Institution talk, she has gone from being a transplant surgeon who saves lives to a transplant surgeon who has the capacity to create life. However, our other motto is 'Compassion, compassion, compassion.' Let us be quite clear that all our efforts are directed at the relief of the suffering of this group of women and their partners.

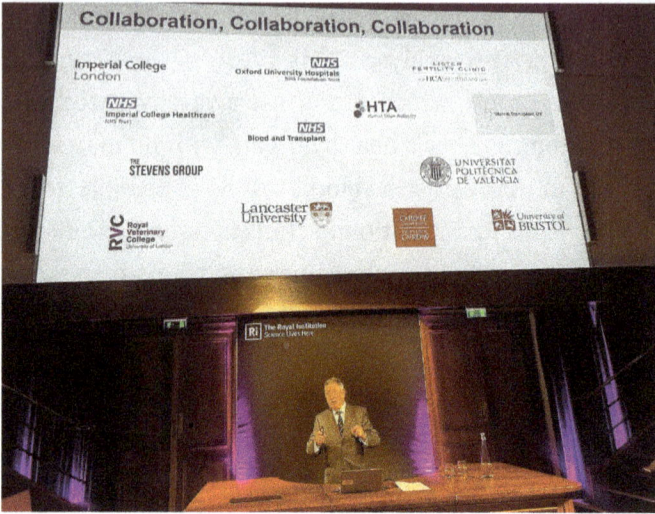

Richard at the Royal Institution below his slide on collaboration.

Our patients have waited long for us to progress these projects over the line, and for them to achieve pregnancy and motherhood. These women have stopped our team from giving up many times over the decades and kept us 'hanging on in there.' We started as a team of gynaecologists – Richard and Srdjan as gynaecological cancer surgeons, Ben and Sal as fertility specialists, and Ari as an obstetrician. Isabel, Venkatesha and Ann started as renal and pancreatic surgeons. This book has tried to tell the story of how this group became one team of uterine transplant surgeons.

The Duke of Wellington's quote with respect to the battle of Waterloo, 'the nearest-run thing you ever saw in your life' bears a striking resemblance to this project!

Epilogue

The team assembled at Queen Charlotte's and Chelsea Hospital in London at 8 am on 27th February 2025. We consisted of obstetricians, gynaecological and transplant surgeons, paediatricians, midwives, and anaesthetists. Miss Bryony Jones, obstetrician, lead the pre-operative huddle of over 20 people — a Queen Charlotte's record number of healthcare professionals in one theatre for one delivery.

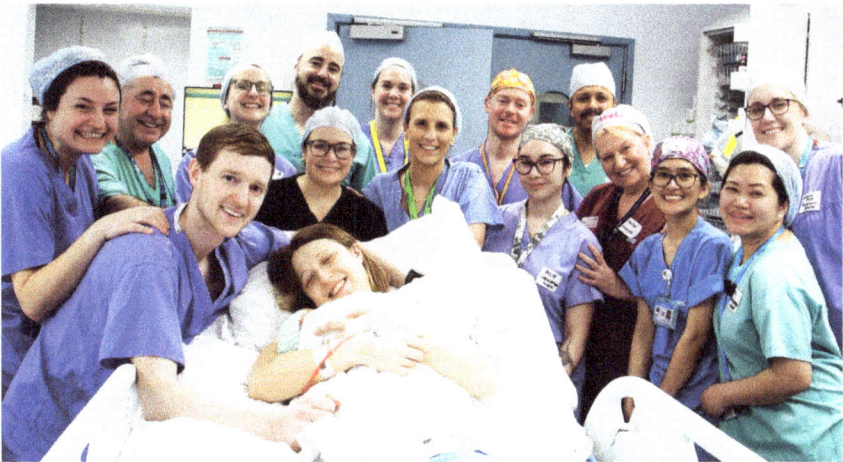

Delivery of a new life.

Later that morning, a beautiful little baby girl weighing 2.1 kg was delivered: the first baby born in the UK following uterine transplantation. This was the culmination of a ten-year journey for Grace and Angus, the parents. There were many tears from all of us in that theatre — so many years of effort, and finally Womb Transplant UK had delivered its first baby.

Incredibly touchingly, halfway through the Caesarean section the parents told us that they had chosen to name the baby Amy Isabel: Amy after Grace's sister who donated her uterus, and Isabel after our Isabel; as Grace said, 'spelt the Spanish way, not the Scottish way, in honour of Isabel.' It is to be hoped that Amy Isabel is the first of many babies to come from our programmes.

Now this is not the end. It is not even the beginning of the end. But it is, perhaps, the end of the beginning.

WS Churchill

Glossary of Terms

anastomosis	connection made surgically between adjacent blood vessels or other channels in the body
anterior	front of the body
arterial	related to arteries
beta HCG	a hormone produced by the placenta in pregnancy
BMI	measurement of leanness based on a person's height and weight
cervix	neck of the womb
double-slinging	placing a sling around the ureter on either side of the uterine arteries and veins
-ectomy	removal of an organ, e.g., appendicectomy
endometrium	layer of tissue lining the uterus
Fallopian tube	'tube' between the uterus and ovary
fibroids	benign growths originating in the uterus
frozen section	type of analysis performed on a tumour

gynaecology	field of medicine treating women's diseases, particularly regarding the reproductive system
haematuria	presence of blood in urine
haemorrhage	loss of blood
heparin	blood thinning medication used to prevent blood clots
histopathology	the diagnosis and study of diseases of the tissues
hysterectomy	surgical removal of the uterus
immunosuppression	suppression of the immune system
inferior epigastric vessels	vessels in the anterior abdominal wall
IVF	a fertility treatment
laparoscopic	keyhole surgery
lymph nodes	glands situated alongside blood vessels
metastasis	cancer which has spread from its primary (original) site, also known as secondary cancer
obstetrics	field of medicine concerned with childbearing
omentum	fatty structure hanging from the large bowel
oncology	field of medicine concerned with diagnosing and treating cancers
-oscopy	to look into an organ, e.g., hysteroscopy: to look into the uterus

-ostomy	to fashion a hole in an organ, e.g., colostomy: to fashion a hole in the colon (large bowel)
ovaries	organs that produce eggs, and cease to function at menopause
parametrium	tissue lying lateral to the cervix
perfusion	passing fluids through the body's circulatory system
peritoneum	membrane surrounding the abdominal organs
primary cancer	place where a cancer has started
pulmonary embolism	blockage in the lungs caused by a blood clot
pulse oximetry	test to measure level of oxygen in the blook
secondary cancer	cancer that has spread from its original, primary site, also known as metastases
stage	extent to which a cancer has spread, written as I, II, III or IV — I being earliest, i.e., not spread, and IV latest, i.e., spread widely
superior vesical vessels	blood vessels supplying the bladder
thrombosis	blood clots
ureters	tube that carries urine from the kidney to the bladder
uterosacral ligaments	supportive band of tissue connecting the uterus to the lower spine

uterus	womb
vagina	tube of muscular tissue and mucosa between the vulva and the cervix
venous	related to veins
VIN	pre-cancerous condition of the vulva
vulva	skin on the outside of the vagina, encompassing the labia majora (hair-bearing skin), the labia minora (the inner lips) and the clitoris, perineum and mons pubis

List of Publications by Womb Transplant UK Relating to Fertility Preservation and Restoration

Ahmed-Salim Y, Galazis N, Bracewell-Milnes T, Phelps DL, Jones BP, Chan M, Munoz-Gonzales MD, Matsuzono T, Smith JR, Yazbek J, Krell J, Ghaem-Maghami S, and Saso S. **Int J Gynecol Cancer**. The application of metabolomics in ovarian cancer management: a systematic review. 2020 May; 31(5): 754–774. https://doi.org/10.1136/ijgc-2020-001862.

Ahmed-Salim Y, Saso S, Meehan HE, Galazis N, Phelps DL, Jones BP, Chan M, Chawla M, Lathouras K, Gabra H, Fotopoulou C, Ghaem-Maghami S, and Smith JR. A novel application of calcium electroporation to cutaneous manifestations of gynaecological cancer. **Eur J Gynaecol Oncol**. 2021; 42(4): 662–672. https://doi.org/10.31083/j.ejgo4204102.

Al-Khatib K, Sieunarine K, Lindsay I, and Smith JR. Metastatic Hurthle cell carcinoma in the abdomen masquerading as a primary ovarian tumour. **Int J Gynecol Cancer**. 2006; 16: 429–432.

Bansal AS, Bora SA, Saso S, Smith JR, Johnson MR, and Thum MY. Mechanism of human chorionic gonadotrophin-mediated immuno-modulation in pregnancy. **Expert Rev Clin Immunol**. 2012; 8(8): 747–753.

Barcroft JF, Galazis N, Jones BP, Getreu N, Bracewell-Milnes T, Grewal KJ, Sorbi F, Yazbek J, Lathouras K, Smith JR, Hardiman P, Thum MY, Ben-Nagi J, Ghaem-Maghami S, Verbakel J, and Saso S. Fertility treatment and cancers-the eternal conundrum: a systematic review and meta-analysis. **Hum Reprod.** 2021 Mar 18; 36(4): 1093–1107. https://doi.org/10.1093/humrep/deaa293.

Bayar E, Williams NJ, Alghrani A, Murugesu S, Saso S, Bracewell-Milnes T, Thum MY, Nicopoullos J, Sangster P, Yasmin E, Smith JR, Wilkinson S, Pacey A, and Jones BP. Fertility preservation and realignment in transgender women. **Hum Fertil (Camb).** 2023 Jul; 26(3): 463–482. https://doi.org/10.1080/14647273.2022.2163195.

Clancy NT, Saso S, Stoyanov D, Sauvage V, Corless DJ, Boyd M, Noakes DE, Thum MY, Ghaem-Maghami S, Smith JR, and Elson DS. Multispectral imaging of organ viability during uterine transplantation surgery in rabbits and sheep. **J Biomed Opt.** 2016; 21(10): 106006. https://doi.org/10.1117/1.JBO.21.10.106006.

Clancy NT, Sauvage V, Elson DS, Saso, S, Stoyanov D, Corless DJ, Boyd M, Noakes DE, Thum MY, Ghaem-Maghami S, and Smith JR. Multispectral imaging of organ viability during uterine transplantation surgery. **Int Soc Opt Eng.** 2014. https://doi.org/10.1117/12.2040518.

Cottrell CM, Ohaegbulam GC, Smith JR, and Del Priore G. Fertility-sparing treatment in cervical cancer: abdominal trachelectomy. **Best Pract Res Clin Obstet Gynaecol.** 2021 Sep; 75: 72–81. https://doi.org/10.1016/j.bpobgyn.2021.01.011.

Del Priore G, Altman MW, Fontaine EM, Ruiz Jr. GE, Smith JR, and Klapper AS. Abdominal trachelectomy modified (ATM) for benign indications. **Fertil Steril.** 2008; 90: 445–446.

Del Priore G, Ghalian RA, Goldfrank DJ, Esdaile BA, Silverstein ML, and Smith JR. Supracervical hysterectomy: a survey of the society of gynaecologic oncologists. **J Obstet Gynaecol.** 2003; 101(4): S59.

Del Priore G, Klapper AS, Gurshumov E, Vargas MM, Ungar L, and Smith JR. Rescue radical trachelectomy for preservation of fertility in benign disease. **Fertil Steril**. 2010; 94: 1910.e5–7.

Del Priore G, Saso S, Meslin E, Tzakis A, Brännström M, Clarke A, Vianna R, Sawyer R, and Smith JR. Uterine transplantation – a real possibility? The Indianapolis consensus. **Hum Reprod**. 2013; 28: 288–291.

Del Priore G, Schlatt S, Wagner R, Smith JR, and Stega J. Primate uterus allograft transplantation. **Fertil Steril**. 2007; 88(1): S221–222.

Del Priore G, Smith JR, and Ungar L. New indication for gravid abdominal radical trachelectomy: cervix cancer during pregnancy. **Obstetrics & Gynecology**. 2006; 107(4): 107S.

Del Priore G, Smith JR, Boyle DC, Corless DJ, Zacharia FB, Noakes DA, Diflo T, Grifo JA, and Zhang JJ. Uterine transplantation, abdominal trachelectomy, and other reproductive options for cancer patients. **Ann N Y Acad Sci**. 2001; 943: 287–295.

Del Priore G, Smith JR, and Ungar L. Radical abdominal trachelectomy at 11 weeks' pregnancy. **Fertil Steril**. 2005; 84(1): S477.

Del Priore G, Stega J, Sieunarine K, Ungar L, and Smith JR. Human uterus retrieval from a multi-organ donor. **Obstet Gynecol**. 2007; 109: 101–104.

Del Priore G, Zhang JJ, Diflo T, Silber S, and Smith JR. Ovary and uterine transplant: a feasible rat model. **Fertil Steril**. 2005; 84(1): S58.

Doumplis D, Al Khatib K, Sieunarine K, Lindsay I, Seckl M, Bridges J, and Smith JR. A review of the management by hysterectomy of 25 cases of gestational trophoblastic tumours from March 1993 to January 2006. **Br J Obstet Gynaecol**. 2007; 114: 1168–1171.

Doumplis D, Majeed G, Sieunarine K, Richardson R, and Smith JR. Adverse effects related to icodextrin 4% – our experience. **Gynecol Surg**. 2007; 4: 97–100.

Esdaile BA, Chalian RA, Del Priore G, and Smith JR. A randomised comparison of total or supracervical hysterectomy: surgical complications and clinical outcomes. **Obstet Gynecol.** 2004; 103: 581.

Esdaile BA, Chalian RA, Del Priore G, and Smith JR. The role of supracervical hysterectomy in benign disease of the uterus. **J Obstet Gynaecol.** 2006; 26: 52–8.

Fulwell L, Taylor-Clarke M, Chatterjee J, Mason P, McIndoe A, Smith JR, Farthing A, and Ghaem-Maghami, S. P1013 Morbidity and mortality associated with the use of inferior vena caval filters prior to major gynaecological oncology surgery in patients with venous thromboembolism: experience at the Hammersmith Hospital, London, UK. **Int J Gyn Obs.** 2009; 107(2): S697.

Galazis N, Saso S, Sorbi F, Jones B, Landolfo C, Al-Memar M, Ben-Nagi J, Smith JR, and Yazbek J. Intraoperative ultrasound during fertility sparing surgery: a systematic review and practical applications. **Gynecol Obstet Invest.** 2020; 85(2): 127–148. https://doi.org/10.1159/000505689. Epub 2020 Jan 22.

Ghorani E, Ramaswami R, Smith RJ, Savage PM, and Seckl MJ. Anti-Müllerian hormone in patients treated with chemotherapy for gestational trophoblastic neoplasia does not predict short-term fertility. **J Reprod Med.** 2016 May–Jun; 61(5–6): 205–209.

Goddard R, Stafford M, and Smith JR. Selective uterine artery ligation. **Br J Obstet Gynaecol.** 1998; 105: 125–128.

Goddard R, Stafford M, and Smith JR. The B-Lynch surgical technique for the control of massive postpartum haemorrhage: an alternative to hysterectomy? Five cases reported. **Br J Obstet Gynaecol.** 1998; 105: 126.

Hurst SA, Del Priore G, Ungar L, and Smith JR. Abdominal radical trachelectomy − A fertility-sparing treatment for cervical cancer. **TOG.** 2010; 12(1): 64–65.

Jones BP, Al-Chami A, Gonzalez X, Arshad F, Green J, Bracewell-Milnes T, Saso S, Smith JR, Serhal P, and Ben-Nagi J. Is oocyte maturity influenced by ovulation trigger type in oocyte donation cycles? **Hum Fertil.** 2021 Dec; 24(5): 360–366. https://doi.org/10.1080/ 14647273.2019.1671614.

Jones BP, Alghrani A, and Smith JR. Re: uterine transplantation in transgender women: medical, legal and ethical considerations. **BJOG.** 2018 Nov 21. https://doi.org/10.1111/1471-0528.15558.

Jones BP, Kasaven L, Vali S, Saso S, Jalmbrant M, Bracewell-Milnes T, Thum MY, Quiroga I, Friend P, Diaz-Garcia C, Ghaem-Maghami S, Yazbek J, Lees C, Testa G, Johannesson L, Jones B, and Smith JR. Uterine transplantation: review of livebirths and reproductive implications. **Transplantation.** 2021 Aug 1; 105(8): 1695–1707. https://doi. org/10.1097/TP.0000000000003578.

Jones BP, Kasaven LS, Chan M, Vali S, Saso S, Bracewell-Milnes T, Thum MY, Nicopoullos J, Diaz-Garcia C, Quiroga I, Yazbek J, and Smith JR. Uterine transplantation in 2021: recent developments and the future. **Clin Obstet Gynecol.** 2022 Mar 1; 65(1): 4–14. https://doi. org/10.1097/GRF.0000000000000680.

Jones BP, L'Heveder A, Saso S, Barcroft J, Richardson R, Kaur B, Ghaem-Maghami S, Yazbek J, and Smith JR. Conservative management of uterine adenosarcoma: lessons learned from 20 years of follow-up. **Arch Gynecol Obstet.** 2019 Nov; 300(5): 1383–1389. https://doi.org/10.1007/s00404-019-05306-6.

Jones BP, L'Heveder, A, Saso S, Yazbek J, Smith JR, and Dooley M. Sports gynaecology. **The Obstetrician & Gynaecologist.** 2019; 21: 85–94. https://doi.org/10.1111/tog.12557.

Jones BP, Rajamanoharan A, Vali S, Williams NJ, Saso S, Thum MY, Ghaem-Maghami S, Quiroga I, Diaz-Garcia C, Thomas P, Wilkinson S, Yazbek J, and Smith JR. Perceptions and motivations for uterus transplant in transgender women. **JAMA Netw Open.** 2021 Jan 4; 4(1): e2034561. https://doi.org/10.1001/jamanetworkopen.2020.34561.

Jones BP, Rajamanoharan A, Williams NJ, Vali S, Saso S, Mantrali I, Jalmbrant M, Thum MY, Diaz-Garcia C, Ghaem-Maghami S, Wilkinson S, Quiroga I, Friend P, Yazbek J, and Smith JR.

Uterine transplantation using living donation: a cross-sectional study assessing perceptions, acceptability, and suitability. **Transplant Direct**. 2021 Feb 18; 7(3): e673. https://doi.org/10.1097/TXD.0000000000001124.

Jones BP, Ranaei-Zamani N, Vali S., Williams N, Saso S, Thum MY, Al-Memar M., Dixon N, Rose G, Testa G, Johannesson L, Yazbek J, Wilkinson S, and Smith JR. Options for acquiring motherhood in absolute uterine factor infertility: adoption, surrogacy and uterine transplantation. **Obstet Gynaecol**. 2021; 23(2): 138–147. https://doi.org/10.1111/tog.12729.

Jones BP, Saso S, and Smith JR. Thinking outside the pelvis: cross-fertilisation learning between specialties. **The Obstetrician & Gynaecologist (TOG)**. Aug 2018. https://doi.org/10.1111/tog.12514.

Jones BP, Saso S, Bracewell-Milnes T, Thum MY, Nicopoullos J, Diaz-Garcia C, Friend P, Ghaem-Maghami S, Testa G, Johannesson L, Quiroga I, Yazbek J, and Smith JR. Human uterine transplantation: a review of outcomes from the first 45 cases. **BJOG**. 2019 Oct; 126(11): 1310–1319. https://doi.org/10.1111/1471-0528.15863. Epub 2019 Aug 13.

Jones BP, Saso S, Farren J, El-Bahrawy M, Ghaem-Maghami S, Smith JR, and Yazbek J. Ultrasound-guided laparoscopic ovarian wedge resection in recurrent serous borderline ovarian tumours. **Int J Gynecol Cancer**. 2017; 27(9): 1813–1818. https://doi.org/10.1097/IGC.0000000000001096.

Jones BP, Saso S, L'Heveder A, Bracewell-Milnes T, Thum MY, Diaz-Garcia C, Quiroga I, Ghaem-Maghami S, Testa G, Johannesson L, MacIntyre D, Bennett P, Yazbek J, and Smith JR. The vaginal microbiome in uterine transplantation. **BJOG**. 2019; 127(2): 230–238. https://doi.org/10.1111/1471-0528.15881.

Jones BP, Saso S, Mania A, Smith JR, Serhal P, and Ben Nagi J. The dawn of a new Ice Age: social egg freezing. **Acta Obstet Gynecol Scand**. 2018 Feb 26. https://doi.org/10.1111/aogs.13335.

Jones BP, Saso S, Yazbek J, and Smith JR. Re: UK criteria for uterus transplantation: a review. **BJOG**. 2019 Nov; 126(12): 1507–1508. https://doi.org/10.1111/1471-0528.15912.

Jones BP, Saso S, Yazbek J, and Smith JR. Uterine transplantation: past, present and future. **BJOG**. 2016; 123(9): 1434–1438. https://doi.org/10.1111/1471-0528.13963.

Jones BP, Saso S, Yazbek J, Thum MY, Quiroga I, Ghaem-Maghami S, Smith JR; Royal College of Obstetricians and Gynaecologists. Uterine Transplantation: Scientific Impact Paper No. 65 April 2021. **BJOG**. 2021 Sep; 128(10): e51–e66. https://doi.org/10.1111/1471-0528.16697.

Jones BP, Saso S, Farren J, El-Bahrawy M, Smith JR, and Yazbek J. Intra-operative ultrasound guided laparoscopic ovarian tissue preserving surgery in the treatment of recurrent borderline ovarian tumors. 2016. **Ultrasound Obstet Gynecol**. Accepted Author Manuscript. https://doi.org/10.1002/uog.17372.

Jones BP, Vali S, Saso S, Devaney A, Bracewell-Milnes T, Nicopoullos J, Thum MY, Kaur B, Roufosse C, Stewart V, Bharwani N, Ogbemudia A, Barnardo M, Dimitrov P, Klucniks A, Katz R, Johannesson L, Diaz-Garcia C, Udupa V, Friend P, Quiroga I, and Smith JR. Living donor uterus transplant in the UK: a case report. **BJOG**. 2023 https://doi.org/10.1111/1471-0528.17639.

Jones BP, Vali S, Saso S, Garcia-Dominguez X, Chan M, Thum MY, Ghaem-Maghami S, Kaur B, García-Valero L, Petrucci L, Yazbek J, Vicente JS, Quiroga I, Marco-Jiménez F, and Smith JR. Endometrial autotransplantation in rabbits: potential for fertility restoration in severe Asherman's syndrome. **Eur J Obstet Gynecol Reprod Biol**. 2020 May; 248: 14–23. https://doi.org/10.1016/j.ejogrb.2020.03.011.

Jones BP, Williams NJ, Saso S, Thum MY, Quiroga I, Yazbek J, Wilkinson S, Ghaem-Maghami S, Thomas P, and Smith JR. Uterine transplantation in transgender women. **BJOG**. 2018 Aug 20. https://doi.org/10.1111/1471-0528.15438.

Kasaven LS, Saso S, Barcroft J, Yazbek J, Joash K, Stalder C, Ben Nagi J, Smith JR, Lees C, Bourne T, and Jones BP. Implications for the future of obstetrics and gynaecology following the COVID-19 pandemic: a commentary. **BJOG.** 2020 Oct; 127(11): 1318–1323. https://doi.org/10.1111/1471-0528.16431.

Kasaven LS, Saso S, Ben Nagi J, Joash K, Yazbek, J, Smith JR, Bourne T, and Jones BP. TOGadvisor: the role of online feedback in obstetrics and gynaecology. **TOG.** 2022; 24: 7–11. https://doi.org/10.1111/tog.12789.

Kuzmin E, Del Priore G, Ungar L, and Smith JR. Uterine transplantation: new hope for infertile women? **Br J Sex Med.** 2008; 30: 7–9.

Kuzmin EY, David A, Simon H, Lindsay I, Noakes D, and Smith JR. Perfusion index, pulse oxymetry and Doppler flow studies to facilitate uterine transplantation. (Abstract ASRM), **Fertil Steril.** 2007; 88: S225.

Lintner B, Saso S, Tarnai L, Novak Z, Palfalvi L, Del Priore G, Smith JR, and Ungar L. Use of abdominal radical trachelectomy to treat cervical cancer greater than 2 cm in diameter. **Int J Gynecol Cancer.** 2013; 23: 1065–1070.

Louis LS, Saso S, Ghaem-Maghami S, Abdalla Y, and Smith JR. The relationship between infertility treatment and cancer including gynaecological cancers. **TOG.** 2013; 15(3): 177–183.

Milingos D, Doumplis D, Savage P, Seckl M, Lindsay I, and Smith JR. Placental site trophoblast tumour with ovarian metastasis. **Int J Gynecol Cancer.** 2007; 17: 925–927.

Milingos D, Doumplis D, Sieunarine K, Savage P, and Smith JR. Uterine arteriovenous malformation: fertility sparing surgery utilizing unilateral ligation of uterine artery and ovarian ligament. **Int J Gynecol Cancer.** 2007; 17: 735–737.

Mitra A, Kindinger L, Kalliala I, Smith JR, Paraskevaidis E, Bennett PR, and Kyrgiou M. Obstetric complications after treatment of cervical intraepithelial neoplasia. **Br J Hosp Med** (Lond). 2016; 77(8): C124–C127. https://doi.org/10.12968/hmed.2016.77.8.C124.

Moxey P, Sieunarine K, Cox J, Lawson AD, Ungar L, and Smith JR. Pulse oximetry and perfusion index measurement to assess uterine perfusion and viability. **Int Surg.** 2006; 91: 223–227.

Nair A, Stega J, Smith JR, and Del Priore G. Uterus transplant: evidence and ethics. **Ann NY Acad Sci.** 2008; 1127: 83–91.

Nair AR, Montemarano N, Gudipudi D, Stega J, Smith JR, and Del Priore G. Potential candidates for uterine transplantation an assessment of need. **Fertil Steril.** 2007; 88(1): S224–225.

Palmieri C, Fisher RA, Sebire NJ, Lindsay I, Smith JR, McCluggage WG, Savage P, and Seckl MJ. Placental site trophoblastic tumour arising from a partial hydatidiform mole. **Lancet.** 2005; 366(9486): 688.

Rakha S, Bayliss C, Sanderson F, Smith JR, Seckl M, and Savage P. Pituitary hCG production and cerebral tuberculosis mimicking disease progression during chemotherapy for an advanced ovarian germ cell tumour. **BMC Cancer.** 2010; 10: 338.

Rockall AG, Qureshi M, Papadopoulou I, Saso S, Butterfield N, Thomassin-Naggara I, Farthing A, Smith JR, and Bharwani N. Role of imaging in fertility-sparing treatment of gynecologic malignancies. **RadioGraphics.** 2016; 36(7): 2214–2233.

Saso S, Bracewell-Milnes T, Ismail L, Hamed AH, Thum MY, Ghaem-Maghami S, Del Priore G, and Smith JR. Psychological assessment tool for patients diagnosed with absolute uterine factor infertility and planning to undergo uterine transplantation. **J Obstet Gynaecol.** 2014; 15: 1–4.

Saso S, Chatterjee J, and Smith JR. Radical trachelectomy: need for a randomized controlled trial? **Acta Obstet Gynaecol Scand.** 2012; 91: 758.

Saso S, Chatterjee J, Georgiou E, Ditri A, Smith JR, and Ghaem-Maghami S. Endometrial cancer – clinical review. **BMJ.** 2012; 343: 84–89.

Saso S, Chatterjee J, Thum Y, Ghaem-Maghami S, Del Priore G, and Smith JR. Pregnancy following allogeneic uterine transplantation in a rabbit model. **Fertil Steril.** 2012; 98(3): 123–124.

Saso S, Chatterjee J, Yazbek J, Thum Y, Keefe KW, Abdallah Y, Naji O, Lindsay I, Savage PM, Seckl MJ, and Smith JR. A case of pregnancy following a modified Strassman procedure applied to treat a placental site trophoblastic tumour. **Br J Obstet Gynaecol.** 2012; 119(13): 1665–1667.

Saso S, Clancy, N, Jones BP, Bracewell-Milnes T, Al-Memar M, Cannon EM, Ahluwalia S, Yazbek J, Thum MY, Bourne T, Elson DS, Smith JR and Ghaem-Maghami S. Use of biomedical photonics in gyneco-logical surgery: a uterine transplantation model. **Future Sci.** 2018 Feb. https://doi.org/10.4155/fsoa-2017-0129.

Saso S, Clarke A, Bracewell-Milnes T, Al-Memar M, Thum MY, Ghaem-Maghami S, Del Priore G, and Smith JR. Survey of perceptions of healthcare professionals in the UK towards uterine transplantation. **Prog Transplant.** 2015; 25(1): 56–63.

Saso S, Clarke A, Bracewell-Milnes T, Saso A, Al-Memar M, Thum M-Y, Yazbek J, Del Priore G, Hardiman P, Ghaem-Maghami S, and Smith JR. Psychological issues associated with absolute uterine factor infertility and attitudes of patients toward uterine transplan-tation, **Prog Transplant.** 2016 26: 28–39, ISSN: 1526–9248.

Saso S, Galazis N, Iacovou C, Kappatou K, Tzafetas M, Jones B, Yazbek J, Lathouras K, Anderson J, Jiao LR, and Smith RJ. Managing growing teratoma syndrome: new insights and clinical applications. **Future Sci OA.** 2019 Oct 10; 5(9): FSO419. https://doi.org/10.2144/fsoa-2019-0075.

Saso S, Ghaem-Maghami S, Chatterjee J, Brewig N, Ungar L, Smith JR, and Del Priore G. Immunology of uterine transplantation: a review. **Reprod Sci.** 2012; 19(2): 123–134.

Saso S, Ghaem-Maghami S, Chatterjee J, Naji O, Farthing A, Mason P, McIndoe A, Hird V, Ungar L, Del Priore G, and Smith JR. Abdominal radical trachelectomy in West London. **Br J Obstet Gynaecol**. 2012; 119: 187–193.

Saso S, Ghaem-Maghami S, Louis LS, Ungar L, Del Priore G, and Smith JR. Uterine transplantation: what else needs to be done before it can become a reality? **J Obs Gynaecol**. 2013; 33: 232–238.

Saso S, Haddad J, Ellis P, Lindsay I Sebire NJ, McIndoe A, Seckl MJ, and Smith JR. Placental site trophoblastic tumours and the concept of fertility preservation. **BJOG**. 2012; 119(3): 369–374.

Saso S, Hamed AH, Docor C, Thum MY, Naji O, Smith JR, Vianna R, and Del Priore G. Is there a role for transplantation in gynaecologic oncology? Autotransplantation and other lessons. **Int J Gynecol Cancer**. 2013; 3: 413–416.

Saso S, Hurst S, Chatterjee J, Kuzmin E, Thum Y, David AL, Hakim N, Corless DJ, Boyd M, Noakes DE, Lindsay I, Ghaem-Maghami S, Del Priore G, and Smith JR. Test of long-term uterine survival after allogeneic transplantation in rabbits. **J Obstet Gynaecol Res**. 2014; 40: 754–762.

Saso S, Jones BP, Bracewell-Milnes T, Huseyin G, Boyle DC, Priore GD, and Smith JR. Gynecological cancers: an alternative approach to healing. **Future Sci OA**. 2017 Jul 12; 3(3): FSO208. https://doi.org/10.4155/fsoa-2017-0022. eCollection 2017 Aug.

Saso S, Logan K, Abdalla Y, Louis LS, Ghaem-Maghami S, Smith JR, and Del Priore G. Use of cyclosporine in uterine transplantation. **J Transplant**. 2012; 134936.

Saso S, Petts G, Chatterjee J, Thum MY, David AL, Corless D, Boyd M, Noakes D, Lindsay I, Del Priore G, Ghaem-Maghami S, and Smith JR. Uterine allotransplantation in a rabbit model using aorto-caval anastomosis: a long-term viability study. **Eur J Obstet Gynecol Reprod Biol**. 2014; 182C: 185–193.

Saso S, Petts G, David AL, Thum MY, Chatterjee J, Vicente JS, Marco-Jimenez F, Corless D, Boyd M, Noakes D, Lindsay I, Del Priore G, Ghaem-Maghami S, and Smith JR. Achieving an early pregnancy following allogeneic uterine transplantation in a rabbit model. **Eur J Obstet Gynecol Reprod Biol.** 2015; 185: 164–169.

Saso S, Petts G, Thum MY, Corless D, Boyd M, Noakes D, Del Priore G, Ghaem-Maghami S, and Smith JR. Achieving uterine auto-transplantation in a sheep model using iliac vessel anastomosis: a short-term viability study. **Acta Obstet Gynecol Scand.** 2015 Mar; 94(3): 245–252.

Saso S, Sawyer R, O'Neill NM, Tzafetas M, Sayasneh A, Hassan Hamed A, Elliott F, Thum MY, Ghaem-Maghami S, Lee MJ, Smith JR, and Del Priore G. Trachelectomy during pregnancy: what has experience taught us? **J Obstet Gynaecol Res.** 2015 Apr; 41(4): 640–645. doi: 10.1111/jog.12594.

Saso S, Tziraki M, Clancy NT, Song L, Bracewell-Milnes T, Jones BP, Al-Memar M, Yazbek J, Thum MY, Sayasneh A, Bourne T, Smith JR, Elson DS, and Ghaem-Maghami S. Use of laser speckle contrast analysis during pelvic surgery in a uterine transplantation model. **Future Sci OA.** 2018 Aug 1; 4(7): FSO324. https://doi.org/10.4155/fsoa-2018-0017.

Savvidou M, Setchell T, Sieunarine K, and Smith JR. Conservative surgical management of ruptured interstitial ectopic pregnancy. **Acta Obstet Gynecol Scand.** 2006; 85: 629–631.

Sienarine K, Ungar L, Smith JR, Lindsay I, Moxey P, Boyle DCM, and Del Priore G. Selective vessel ligation in the pelvis: an invaluable tool in certain surgical procedures. **Int J Gynecol Cancer.** 2006; 15: 967–973.

Sieunarine K, Boyle DCM, Corless DJ, Noakes DE, Ungar L, Marr CE, Lindsay I, Del Priore G, and Smith JR. Pelvic vascular prospects for uterine transplantation. **Int Surg.** 2006; 91: 217–222.

Sieunarine K, Corless DJ, Noakes DE, Ungar L, Del Priore G, and Smith JR. Fertility restoration – uterine transplantation using a macrovascular patch technique. **Fertil Steril.** 2005; 84(1): S477–S478.

Sieunarine K, Cowie A, Bartlett J, Lindsay I, and Smith JR. A novel approach in the management of a recurrent adenomatoid tumour of the uterus utilizing a Strassman technique. **Int J Gynecol Cancer.** 2005; 15: 671–675.

Sieunarine K, Doumplis D, Kuzmin E, Corless DJ, Hakim N, Del Priore G, and Smith JR. Uterine allotransplantation in the rabbit using a macrovascular patch. **Int Surg.** 2009; 93: 288–294.

Sieunarine K, Hakim N, Corless DJ, Noakes DE, Ungar L, Del Priore G, and Smith JR. Is it feasible to use a large vessel patch with a uterine allograft en bloc for uterine transplantation? **Int Surg.** 2005; 90: 257–261.

Sieunarine K, Lawton F, and Smith JR. Chronic pelvic pain: a rare complication following a LLETZ. **Int J Gynecol Cancer.** 2006; 16: 620–622.

Sieunarine K, Lindsay I, Ungar L, Del Priore G, and Smith JR. Cold ischaemic preservation of human uterine tissue. **Int Surg.** 2008; 93: 366–372.

Sieunarine K, Noakes D, Smith E, Smith JR, Ungar L, Hakim N, Corless D, and Del Priore G. Is it feasible to use a large vessel patch with a uterine allograft en bloc for uterine transplantation. **Int Surg.** 2006; 90: 257–261.

Sieunarine K, Zakaria F, Boyle DCM, Corless DJ, Noakes DE, Lindsay I, Lawson A, Ungar L, Del Priore G, and Smith JR. Possibilities for fertility restoration − a new surgical technique. **Int Surg.** 2005; 90: 257–261.

Smith JR, Boyle D, Corless D, Lawson A, McColl J, Ungar L, Del Priore G, and Bridges J. Abdominal radical trachelectomy: a new approach to the management of early cervical cancer. **Br J Obstet Gynaecol.** 1997; 104: 1196–1200.

Smith JR, Ghaem-Maghami S, McIndoe A, Farthing A, Mason P, Ungar L, and Del Priore G. Fertility-sparing surgery for young women with early-stage cervical cancer. **Br J Obstet Gynaecol.** 2011; 377–378.

Smith JR, Hurst SA, Kuzmin E, Noakes D, Corless D, and Del Priore G. Successful uterine transplantation in the rabbit model. **Fertil Steril.** 2009; 92(3).

Ungar L, Palfalvi L, Hogg R, Siklos P, Boyle DC, Del Priore G, and Smith JR. Abdominal radical trachelectomy: a fertility-preserving option for women with cervical cancer. **Br J Obstet Gynaecol.** 2005; 112: 366–369.

Ungar L, Smith JR, Pálfalvi L, and Del Priore G. Abdominal radical trachelectomy during pregnancy to preserve pregnancy and fertility. **Obstet Gynecol.** 2006; 108: 811–814.

Vali S, Jones BP, Saso S, Fertleman M, Testa G, Johanesson L, Alghrani A, and Smith JR. Uterine transplantation: legal and regulatory implications in England. **BJOG.** 2021 Sep 17. https://doi.org/10.1111/1471-0528.16927.

Vali S, Jones BP, Saso S, and Smith JR. The impact of COVID-19 on the motivations of women seeking a uterus transplant. **Future Sci OA.** 2023 28; 9(2): FSO846. https://doi.org/10.2144/fsoa-2022-0047.

Vali S, Jones BP, Saso S, Yazbek J, Quiroga I, and Smith JR. Uterus transplantation: a 50-year journey. **Clin Obs Gyn.** 2021 Dec 29.

Vali S, Jones BP, Sheikh S, Saso S, Quiroga I, and Smith JR. Attitudes, knowledge, and perceptions among women toward uterus transplantation and donation in the UK. **Front Med (Lausanne).** 2023 Aug 16; 10: 1223228. https://doi.org/10.3389/fmed.2023.1223228.

Wahba J, Natoli M, Whilding L, Smith JR, Maher J, and Ghaem-Maghami S. Synergistic immuno-chemotherapy for ovarian cancer, **BJOG.** 2016; 123: E6–E7, ISSN: 1470-0328.

Wahba J, Natoli M, Whilding LM, Parente-Pereira AC, Jung Y, Zona S, Lam EW, Smith JR, Maher J, and Ghaem-Maghami S. Chemotherapy-induced apoptosis, autophagy and cell cycle arrest are key drivers of synergy in chemo-immunotherapy of epithelial ovarian cancer. **Cancer Immunol Immunother.** 2018 Nov; 67(11): 1753–1765.

Wali S, Chatterjee J, Zeegen R, and Smith JR. Concealed haematometra causing chronic upper abdominal pain. **J Obstet Gynaecol**. 2014; 30: 1–2.

Wang J, Papanastasopoulos P, Savage P, Smith JR, Fisher C, and El-Bahrawy MA. A unique case of extraovarian sex-cord stromal fibrosarcoma, with subsequent relapse of differentiated sex-cord tumor. **Int J Gynecol Pathol**. 2015; 34(4): 363–368.

Zakaria F, Boyle D, Del Priore G, Corless D, Ungars L, and Smith JR. Uterine transplant: a successful porcine model. **Fertil Steril**. 2001; 76(1): S106.

Books that Support Womb Transplant UK

Smith JR, Del Priore G. *Women's Cancers: Pathways to Living*. Imperial College Press (now World Scientific), London, UK, 2015.

Smith JR. *The Journey: Spirituality, Pilgrimage, Chant*. Darton Longman and Todd, London, UK, 2016.

Smith JR. *A Very Byzantine Journey*. Sacristy Press, Durham, UK, 2022.

Smith JR. *Cancer and Infertility: A Story of Hope*. Mensch Publishing, London, UK, 2023.

Smith JR, Koustsouvelis V, Smith L, Smith M, Koutsouvelis T. *The Monymusk Reliquary: The Brecbennach of St Columba*. JRSmith Healthcare, London, UK, 2024.

All titles are available on Amazon.

www.ingramcontent.com/pod-product-compliance
Lightning Source LLC
Chambersburg PA
CBHW061248220326
41599CB00028B/5566